The Best of
THANKSGIVING

80+ Recipes and Inspiration for a festive holiday meal

ANGELA MAYS

Copyright © 2024 by Angela Mays

All rights reserved.

No portion of this book may be reproduced in any form without written permission from the publisher or author.

Table of Contents

Thanksgiving Formulas 5
How to Create Cornbread Dressing 7
What Temperature to Cook a Turkey 10
Can You Solidify Mashed Potatoes? 16
How to Form Green Beans Almondine 19
Turkey Pot Pie 22
Nectar Cornbread 30
Old-Fashioned Scalloped Corn 31
New or Canned Pumpkin in Pumpkin Pie 35
Does Pumpkin Pie Got to Be Refrigerated? 37
Best Green Bean Casserole 40
Turkey Giblet Sauce Ingredients 46
Squashed Potato Au Gratin 51
Yummy Sweet Potato Casserole 56
Butter Flaky Pie Outside 61
Sweet Potato Dump Cake Ingredients 79
Apple Pie Ingredients 84
New Cranberry Sauce 91
Butternut Squash Cheesecake 94
Bacon-Garlic Green Beans 98
Sodden and Savory Stuffing 100
Damp vs. Dry Brine 109

Fiery chicken & avocado wraps 115

Firm destroyed chicken 117

Panuozzo sandwich..................................121

Bulgur & quinoa lunch bowls 129

Extreme chorizo ciabatta 132

Egg & rocket pizzas 137

Lime pickle rarebit................................140

Falafel burgers................................142

Prawn & mango serving of mixed greens............146

Chorizo & chickpea soup 147

Classic waffles................................152

Chocolate orange waffles 154

Tomato & pasta soup 161

Spaghetti puttanesca................................167

Coconut angle curry & rice 169

Lemon & greens pesto pasta 176

Pork & apple burgers................................181

Kedgeree with poached egg.......................189

Small fiery veggie pies 197

Italian vegetable soup................................205

Tofu & spinach cannelloni........................226

American hotcakes 237

Chocolate-orange French toast 246

**Thanksgiving Formulas
Cornbread Dressing Fixings**

This convention, which marks the begin of Christmas celebrations, comes from an ancient parade performed by olive-oil mill operators, who utilized to put fire to the wicker strainer mats utilized to press the olives as an act of thanksgiving to the Heavenly Shepherdess (Virgin Mary) for the collect gotten.

Within the Joined Together States, Thanksgiving or Thanksgiving Day may be an open occasion on the fourth Thursday in November. It was initially a day when individuals celebrated the conclusion of the collect and expressed gratitude toward God for it.

This dressing formula comes together rapidly with straightforward fixings. Here's what you'll require:

Cornbread:

This formula begins with disintegrated cornbread. You'll purchase pre-made cornbread, make it from a blend, or make a from-scratch cornbread formula.

Vegetables:

You'll require diced onions and celery.

Butter:

Butter is utilized to saute the new vegetables.

Eggs:

Two eggs include dampness and lavishness. They also act as an authoritative specialist, which implies they offer assistance hold the dressing together.

Stock:

Utilize store-bought or hand crafted chicken stock for more flavor and dampness.

Seasonings:

This cornbread dressing is seasoned with dried sage, salt, and dark pepper. Of course, you'll adjust the seasonings to taste.

How to Create Cornbread Dressing
You'll discover the total, step-by-step formula underneath — but here's a brief outline of what you'll be able anticipate once you make this top-rated cornbread dressing:

Sauté the vegetables in butter until delicate.

Include the sautéed vegetables to the disintegrated cornbread.

Blend within the remaining fixings and blend until well-combined.

Exchange the dressing to an arranged heating dish and heat until brilliant brown.

Fixings

3 mugs crumbled cornbread

2 tablespoons butter

1 little onion, diced

½ container chopped celery

2 huge eggs, beaten

2 mugs chicken stock

1 tablespoon dried sage, or more to taste

salt and ground dark pepper to taste

Juicy Thanksgiving Turkey

This turkey recipe has the control to shape or break your Thanksgiving supper. Fortunately, it's not that difficult to cook an impeccably sodden and flavorful feathered creature! This Thanksgiving turkey recipe couldn't be more cherished by the All recipes community —

reviewers say they come back to it year after year.

each 5 pounds of meat. If you have a 15-pound frozen turkey, it'll take approximately three days to thaw completely within the fridge.

How to Season a Turkey

This flavorful, succulent Thanksgiving turkey is prepared from the interior out:

The depression is stuffed with an herbaceous blend of dried parsley, rosemary, sage, thyme, lemon-pepper flavoring, and salt. The Champagne and chicken broth, which are poured over the turkey some time recently simmering to keep the meat inconceivably damp and delicious, moreover include overwhelming flavor.

What Temperature to Cook a Turkey

If you take after this formula with a 15-pound turkey, your Thanksgiving centerpiece ought to be completely cooked after around 3.5 hours in a stove preheated to 350 degrees F.

How Long to Cook a Turkey

We suggest cooking an unstuffed turkey for almost 13-15 minutes per pound. This 15-pound turkey should be completely cooked inside around 3.5 hours — but you ought to continuously check the inside temperature some time recently serving to anticipate nourishment harming.

What Temperature Is Turkey Done?

An instant-read thermometer inserted into the thickest part of the thigh, close the bone, ought to examine at least 180 degrees F.

How to Carve a Turkey?

Carving a turkey isn't as troublesome as you might think You'll simply require a cut, a cutting board, a meat fork, and a couple simple to-follow edifying. That's where we come in! Check out our step-by-step turkey carving direct (with photographs!) to memorize all around the surprisingly simple handle.

Fixings

2 tablespoons dried parsley

2 tablespoons ground dried rosemary

2 tablespoons rubbed dried sage

2 tablespoons dried thyme takes off

1 tablespoon lemon-pepper flavoring

1 tablespoon salt

1 (15 pound) entire turkey, neck and giblets evacuated

1 medium orange, cut into 8 wedges

1 medium onion, chopped into expansive pieces

1 medium carrot, cut into 1/2-inch cuts

2 stalks celery, cut into 1/2-inch cuts

1 (750 milliliter) bottle champagne

1 (14.5 ounce) can chicken broth

Headings

Assemble all fixings. Preheat the oven to 350 degrees F (175 degrees C). Line a roaster with sheets of aluminum thwart long enough to wrap around turkey.

Blend parsley, rosemary, sage, thyme, lemon-pepper seasoning, and salt together in a little bowl.

Rub herb mixture into turkey depth, then stuff with orange wedges, onion, carrot, and celery. Tie turkey legs beside kitchen string, at that point tuck the wings beneath the body.

Put turkey on the thwart within the simmering dish. Pour champagne and chicken broth over turkey, making beyond any doubt to induce a few fluids within the depression.

Bring aluminum thwart up and over the best of turkey and seal; try to keep the thwart from touching the turkey.

Broil turkey within the preheated broiler until juices run clear, 2 ½ to 3 hours. Reveal turkey and proceed heating until the skin turns brilliant brown, 30 to 60 more minutes. An instant-read thermometer embedded into the thickest portion of thigh, close the bone, ought to examine 180 degrees F (82 degrees C).

Evacuate turkey from the stove, cover with two sheets of aluminum thwart, and permit to rest in a warm region some time recently cutting, 10 to 15 minutes.

Fundamental Pounded Potatoes

How to Create Squashed Potatoes

You'll discover the total, step-by-step recipe below — but here's a brief outline of what you'll be able anticipate after you make these squashed potatoes:

Bubble the potatoes:

Include the potatoes and garlic to an expansive pot of salted, bubbling water. Diminish the warm and stew until the potatoes are delicate.

Warm the drain:

Warm the drain and butter in a pan until the butter is dissolved.

Pound the potatoes:

Deplete the potatoes, at that point return them to the pot. Gradually include the warm drain blend, pounding with a potato masher or blending with a blender until the potatoes are smooth and rich. Season to taste.

How Long to Bubble Potatoes for Pounded Potatoes?

Peeled and quartered potatoes ought to be impeccably bubbled after approximately 15-20 minutes. In case you take off your potatoes entirety, it'll take a bit longer.

How to Store Squashed Potatoes

Permit the pounded potatoes to cool totally, at that point exchange them to an airtight container. Store within the fridge for three to four days. Warm in the microwave, within the broiler, or on the stove.

Can You Solidify Mashed Potatoes?
Yes, you'll be able solidify pounded potatoes in single or group servings for up to one month. Defrost them within the cooler overnight or warm them from-frozen within the moderate cooker, on the stove, or within the stove.

Fixings

2 pounds heating potatoes, peeled and quartered

3 cloves garlic, peeled, or to taste (Discretionary)

1 glass drain

2 tablespoons butter

salt and ground dark pepper to taste

Directions

Bring an expansive pot of salted water to a bubble. Include potatoes and garlic, lower warm to medium, and stew until potatoes are delicate, 15 to 20 minutes.

When the potatoes are nearly wrapped up, warm drain and butter in a little saucepan over moo warm until butter is liquefied.

Deplete potatoes and return to the pot. Gradually include warm drain blend, mixing it in with a potato masher or electric mixer until potatoes are smooth and rich. Season with salt and pepper.

Green Beans Almondine

What Is Green Beans Almondine?

Green beans almondine (a.k.a. amandine) is a French dish that comprises of green beans cooked in spread and flavors, by then finished off with toasted fragmented almonds. It sounds favor, but it's surprisingly basic to create this amazing dish at home with fair a number of essential fixings.

Green Beans Almondine Fixings

These are the straightforward fixings you'll have to be make this green beans almondine formula:

Green beans:

A pound of new green beans ought to make about four servings of green beans almondine.

Slivered almonds:

You'll require 1 ½ ounces (around 6 ½ tablespoons) of slivered almonds.

Butter:

Two tablespoons of butter loans abundance, dampness, and flavor.

Seasonings:

This greens beans almondine formula is flavored with fresh garlic, salt, and pepper.

How to Form Green Beans Almondine
You'll discover the total, step-by-step formula below — but here's a brief outline of what you can expect once you make hand crafted green beans almondine:

Microwave the green beans according to the point by point instructions in Step 1.

Toast the almonds on the stove, expel from heat, and include butter to dissolve.

Return to warm, add garlic and green beans, and season.

Cook until heated through.

How to Store Green Beans Almondine

Store your extra green beans almondine in an airtight container within the fridge for up to three days. Warm on the stove or delicately within the microwave.

Fixings

1 pound new green beans

1 ½ ounces slivered almonds

2 tablespoons butter

2 cloves garlic, minced, or more to taste

salt and ground dark pepper to taste

Headings

Put beans into a microwave-safe casserole dish with sufficient water to cover the foot. Microwave on tall control until almost tender, 8 to 10 minutes. Deplete in a colander and revive beneath cold running water to keep the decent green color.

Heat a frying skillet over medium warm. Include almonds and cook until just beginning to turn brilliant, about 3 to 5 minutes, observing closely so as to not burn. Take pan off of warm and add butter to dissolve. Return to warm and include garlic. Blend in green beans, season with salt and pepper, and continue to stir until warmed through, 3 to 5 minutes.

Turkey Pot Pie
Turkey Pot Pie Fixings

These are the fixings you'll require to make this easy turkey pot pie formula:

Solidified vegetables:

From the cooler walkway, you'll require solidified peas and carrots and solidified green beans.

New vegetables:

From the deliver area, you'll require celery and an onion.

Butter:

The turkey pot pie filling begins with ⅔ container softened butter.

Flour:

All-purpose flour makes a difference make a roux.

Seasonings:

Season the flavorful turkey pot pie with salt, pepper, celery seed, onion powder, and Italian flavoring.

Broth:

Utilize store-bought or custom made chicken broth.

Drain:

Drain is basic to a rich, thick roux.

Turkey:

This turkey pot pie recipe is the culminate way to use leftover cooked turkey.

Cake outsides:

Utilize a store-bought or homemade double crust pastry.

How to Form Turkey Pot Pie?

You'll discover the full, step-by-step formula below — but here's a brief diagram of what you can anticipate when you make this custom made turkey pot pie:

Bubble the solidified vegetables with the celery until the celery is tender.

Cook the onion in butter, at that point whisk within the flour and seasonings until a glue shapes.

Whisk within the chicken broth and drain. Cook, whisking continually, until thick.

Blend the cooked, depleted veggies and turkey to the filling.

Fit cake coverings into two pie dishes. Fill the coverings, at that point cover with the remaining coverings.

Cut little openings into the best of each outside and put the pies on a baking sheet.

Heat, agreeing to the point by point informational in Step 7, until the crusts are golden brown and the filling is bubbly.

You'll effortlessly plan this turkey pie ahead of time. Here's are some make ahead tips from test kitchen experts:

Cover pie with plastic wrap and then aluminum thwart.

When prepared to heat, remove plastic wrap and foil.

Cover the edge of the hull with aluminum foil or a pie outside shield.

Bake at 400 degrees F for 1 hour and 15 minutes.

Uncover and continue to prepare until the outsides are brilliant brown and the filling is bubbly, almost 15 to 20 minutes. The inner temperature of the filling ought to be at least 160 degrees F.

Fixings

2 mugs solidified peas and carrots

2 glasses solidified green beans

1 glass cut celery

2/3 glass butter

2/3 glass chopped onion

2/3 container all-purpose flour

1 teaspoon salt

1 teaspoon ground dark pepper

1/2 teaspoon celery seed

1/2 teaspoon onion powder

1/2 teaspoon Italian seasoning

1 (14 1/2 ounce) can chicken broth

1 1/2 mugs drain

4 cups cubed remaining cooked turkey

2 (14.1 ounce) packages rolled refrigerated unbaked pie hull

Headings

Assemble fixings. Preheat the broiler to 425 degrees F (220 degrees C)

Put solidified peas, carrots, and beans in a medium pot with celery. Include sufficient water to cover and bring to a bubble. Decrease warm to medium-low and stew until celery is delicate, around 5 minutes. Deplete.

Whereas the vegetables are stewing, soften butter in a huge pan over medium warm. Include onion and cook until translucent, around 5 minutes. Include flour, salt, pepper, celery seed, onion powder, and Italian flavoring and whisk until a glue shapes, around 1 diminutive.

Gradually whisk in chicken broth and after that drain until joined. Bring to a stew and cook, whisking always, until sauce thickens, 3 to 5 minutes. Evacuate thickened sauce from the warm. Include cooked, depleted vegetables and cubed turkey and blend until filling is well combined.

Set out two 9-inch pie dishes. Fit 1 pie outside circular into the foot of each dish.

Spoon half of the pot pie filling into each dish, at that point lay the remaining piecrust circular over beat.

Squeeze and roll the beat and foot coverings together at the edges to seal, cutting off any hull hanging over the edge.

Utilize a sharp cut to cut a few little openings in each best outside to permit steam to discharge whereas cooking. Put pies on heating sheets. Cover edge of hull with aluminum thwart or a pie outside shield.

Heat within the preheated stove for 30 minutes. Reveal and proceed to heat until the outsides are brilliant brown and the filling is bubbly, 10 to 15 minutes more. Expel from the stove and cool for 10 minutes some time recently serving.

Nectar Cornbread
Fixings

1 container all-purpose flour

1 glass yellow cornmeal

¼ glass white sugar

1 tablespoon preparing powder

1 glass overwhelming cream

2 huge eggs, delicately beaten

¼ glass vegetable oil

¼ glass nectar

Bearings

Preheat the broiler to 400 degrees F (200 degrees C). Gently oil a 9x9-inch preparing dish.

Mix together flour, cornmeal, sugar, and preparing powder in an expansive bowl; frame a well within the center. Include cream, eggs, oil, and nectar; mix until well combined. Pour hitter into the arranged preparing pan.

Prepare within the preheated broiler until a toothpick embedded into the center comes out clean, 20 to 25 minutes.

Old-Fashioned Scalloped Corn
Fixings

3 (15 ounce) cans cream-style corn

1 glass smashed saltine wafers, separated

½ container butter, softened, separated

2 expansive eggs

½ teaspoon paprika

¼ teaspoon ground dark pepper

Bearings

Preheat the broiler to 350 degrees F (175 degrees C). Butter an 8x11x2-inch casserole dish.

Combine creamed corn, 1/2 container saltine pieces, 1/4 container dissolved butter, and eggs in an expansive bowl; blend well. Pour blend into the arranged dish.

Blend remaining 1/2 glass saltine scraps and remaining 1/4 glass liquefied butter with paprika and pepper in a little bowl. Sprinkle piece topping over casserole.

Heat within the preheated broiler until topping browns somewhat and filling bubbles along edges, 30 to 40 minutes.

Culminate Pumpkin Pie

We have over 130 formulas for hand crafted pumpkin pie here at Allrecipes, but this formula takes the cake (or pie) with over 2,600 five-star evaluations. And its verification that a good recipe doesn't necessarily have to be be a complicated one — you get a great result with canned pumpkin puree and store-bought pie hull. Of course, you'll customize it to suit your inclinations by utilizing new pumpkin or a hand crafted pie outside for that from-scratch taste. Plus, it can be made ahead of time and refrigerated (or frozen) until you're prepared to serve! Your rummage around for the idealize pumpkin pie closes here.

How to Form Pumpkin Pie?

Here's what we cherish around this formula:

This pie is fantastically receptive, indeed for amateur pastry specialists. You'll discover the complete, step-by-step formula underneath — but here's a brief outline of what you'll anticipate:

Make the filling.

Pour the blend into the hull.

Heat for 15 minutes, at that point reduce the warm and proceed heating.

Do You Wish to Daze Prepare the Pie Outside?

Daze preparing alludes to preparing pie hull, either in part or completely, without filling it. Why would you be doing this? Pie with a custard-based filling, such as pumpkin, generally requires little broiler time, which implies you will need to allow your crust a bit of a head begin to ensure you do not conclusion up with a raw, saturated foot.

A few reviewers suggest blind preparing the pie hull within the recipe, particularly in the event that you're employing a hand crafted pie outside. Learn step-by-step how to blind bake a pie outside, whether store-bought or hand crafted. In case you're employing a solidified pie hull, you can frequently discover enlightening for blind heating on the bundle.

New or Canned Pumpkin in Pumpkin Pie
Note that this formula calls for canned pumpkin, not "pumpkin pie filling," which is as of now spiced. On the off chance that you arrange to utilize the flavors and sweeteners called for in this formula, go for unflavored canned pumpkin.

Whereas there's no disgrace in utilizing canned pumpkin, a few people lean toward the flavor and satisfaction you get from utilizing new pumpkin. In case that's you, use this formula for making pumpkin puree from scratch. A 1 ½-pound pumpkin yields around 2 mugs pounded pumpkin, the same as a 15-ounce can of pumpkin puree.

Can You Employ Pumpkin Pie Flavor

Several reviewers call out using ready-made pumpkin pie flavor — a combination of ground cinnamon, ginger, allspice, nutmeg, and now and then cloves and mace — and extra cinnamon in place of the flavors called for:

"I followed a recommendation that somebody else had made and utilized 2 teaspoon of pumpkin pie zest and 2 teaspoon of ground cinnamon instep," says commentator Devin. Some people lean toward the taste of the store-bought pumpkin pie zest to the person flavors, but ultimately it's a matter of individual inclination (and comfort!).

Does Pumpkin Pie Got to Be Refrigerated?

Yes, pumpkin pie should be put away within the fridge as it is an "egg wealthy pie," concurring to the USDA. Do permit your pie sufficient time to cool some time recently refrigerating it (this will too provide the filling time to set), but do not take off it out at room temperature for more than 2 hours, something else there's a hazard of bacteria development. Pumpkin pie will last up to three to four days within the fridge. If you arrange to form pumpkin pie in advance, we'd recommend making it one to two days in advance and refrigerating — this way you'll still have a couple days for remains, as well!

Can You Solidify Pumpkin Pie?

Custard-based pies solidify astoundingly well, so you'll completely make pumpkin pie ahead of time and solidify it for up to one month in development (hi, stress-free occasions). On the off chance that you go this course, we do recommend heating your pie in an aluminum pie dish.

To solidify pumpkin pie, prepare your pie and permit it to cool totally. At that point wrap it in a few layers of plastic wrap, and take after with an extra layer of aluminum thwart. Solidify for up to one month. When you're prepared to serve, evacuate the aluminum thwart and allow the pie to defrost overnight within the fridge.

How to Create Whipped Cream for Pumpkin Pie

Split pie? Whipped cream to the protect! Utilize hand crafted or store-bought whipped cream with a sprinkle of cinnamon to cover any blemishes on your pie. To form hand crafted whipped cream, take after this top-rated whipped cream formula.

Fixings

1 (15 ounce) can pumpkin puree

1 (14 ounce) can Falcon Brand Sweetened Condensed Drain

2 expansive eggs

1 teaspoon ground cinnamon

½ teaspoon ground ginger

½ teaspoon ground nutmeg

½ teaspoon salt

1 (9 inch) unbaked pie outside

Bearings

Accumulate all fixings and preheat the stove to 425 degrees F (220 degrees C).

Whisk pumpkin puree, condensed drain, eggs, cinnamon, ginger, nutmeg, and salt together in a medium bowl until smooth.

Pour into hull.

Heat within the preheated broiler for 15 minutes.

Diminish stove temperature to 350 degrees F (175 degrees C) and proceed heating until a cut embedded 1 inch from the hull comes out clean, 35 to 40 minutes. Let cool some time recently serving

Best Green Bean Casserole
This green bean casserole is really the leading. Made with just four budget-friendly fixings, you'll come back to this green bean casserole formula year after year.

Green Bean Casserole Fixings

Accept it or not, you'll require fair four fixings to create this classic green bean casserole:

Green beans:

This simple green bean casserole begins with two depleted cans of green beans.

Canned soup:

A can of condensed cream of mushroom soup makes a rich surface and includes savory flavor.

Cheese:

This formula calls for destroyed Cheddar cheese. Utilize sharp, mellow, or a mix of both.

French-fried onions:

The green bean casserole gets its crunch from a French-fried onion topping.

Discretionary ingredients:

Disintegrated bacon, sautéed mushrooms or onions, garlic, Parmesan cheese, dark pepper

How to Form Green Bean Casserole

You'll discover the total, step-by-step recipe underneath — but here's a brief diagram of what you can anticipate after you make this top-rated green bean casserole:

Blend the beans and soup in a microwave-safe bowl and microwave until warm.

Mix in half the cheese. Microwave until softened and well-blended.

Exchange to a arranged preparing dish. Beat with browned onions and remaining cheese.

Heat in the preheated stove until the cheese is dissolved and the onions are brown.

How Long to Cook Green Bean Casserole?

In a stove preheated to 350 degrees F, this canned green bean casserole ought to be superbly cooked in approximately 10 minutes. Of course, that doesn't incorporate the 5-8 minutes the fixings spend within the microwave!

Can You Make Green Bean Casserole Ahead of Time?

Yes! You'll be able heat this green bean casserole up to three days in progress. Cook it agreeing to the formula, but take off off the French-fried onions. Allow it cool, cover firmly with thwart, and refrigerate until you're prepared to eat.

Fixings

2 (14.5 ounce) cans green beans, depleted

1 (10.5 ounce) can condensed cream of mushroom soup

1 glass destroyed Cheddar cheese, isolated

1 (6 ounce) can French-fried onions

Headings

Preheat the stove to 350 degrees F (175 degrees C).

Blend green beans and condensed soup together in a huge microwave-safe bowl until well combined. Microwave on tall until warm, 3 to 5 minutes.

Mix 1/2 container Cheddar cheese into the green bean blend. Microwave on tall for 2 to 3 minutes.

Exchange blend to a casserole dish and spread equally over the foot. Sprinkle French-fried onions over beat, at that point sprinkle with remaining Cheddar.

Heat within the preheated broiler until cheese is dissolved and the onions are fair turning brown, around 10 minutes.

Turkey Giblet Sauce

Make the foremost of your fowl with this turkey giblet sauce formula. Not a single portion will go to squander!!

Turkey Giblet Sauce Ingredients
These are the fixings you'll have to be make homemade turkey giblet sauce:

· **Giblets:**

You'll require the neck of a turkey and a bundle of turkey giblets (barring the liver).

· **Water:**

Use four glasses of water to bubble the giblets. Blend ½ container of cold water with cornstarch to make a slurry.

· **Cornstarch:**

Cornstarch is blended with cold water to form a slurry, which thickens the sauce.

· **Drippings:**

Turkey drippings, the juices cleared out within the skillet after the turkey has been cooked, have tons of flavor.

· **Egg:**

A chopped hard-boiled egg includes flavor and surface. You'll be able take off it out on the off chance that you'd like a smoother sauce.

· **Seasonings:**

This turkey giblet sauce is basically prepared with fair salt and pepper.

How to Form Turkey Giblet Sauce?

You'll discover a full, step-by-step recipe underneath — but here's a brief outline of what you'll anticipate once you make this delicious turkey giblet gravy:

- **Make the broth:**

Put the giblets and neck in a pot, at that point cover with four mugs of water. Bring to a bubble, decrease the heat, and stew until the broth has decreased by around one container. Strain the broth and reserve around ½ container of the giblets.

- 2. **Thicken with a slurry:**

Whisk the cornstarch and ½ cup of cold water in a little bowl until smooth. Combine the broth and drippings in a pan over medium warm, whisk within the slurry, and bring to a bubble.

- 3. Wrap up the sauce:

Decrease the warm to moo, at that point mix within the chopped giblets and hard-boiled egg. Season with salt and pepper. Stew until the sauce is thickened.

How to Store Turkey Giblet Sauce

Exchange the cooled sauce to a sealed shut holder. Store within the fridge for up to two days. Warm on the stove for the finest comes about.

Can You Solidify Turkey Giblet Sauce?

Exchange the cooled sauce to zip-top cooler packs (or another freezer-safe holder). Wrap in thwart for included security against cooler burn. Lay flat within the cooler and utilize inside four months. Defrost within the cooler overnight, at that point warm on the stove.

Fixings

1 bundle of giblets and neck from turkey, barring liver

4 mugs water

1 container turkey drippings

½ glass cold water

6 tablespoons cornstarch

1 expansive hard-cooked egg, chopped

salt and ground dark pepper to taste

Bearings

Assemble all fixings.

Combine turkey giblets, neck, and 4 mugs water in a pot; bring to a bubble. Diminish warm to moo and stew until broth is decreased to 3 glasses, around 1 hour.

Strain broth and save 1/2 glass giblets.

Combine strained broth and turkey drippings in a pan over medium heat. Whisk together 1/2 container cold water and cornstarch in a little bowl until smooth; pour into broth blend within the pan and bring to a bubble.

Whereas broth is coming to a bubble, finely chop giblets.

Diminish warm to low; blend giblets and hard-cooked egg into sauce.

Stew until sauce is thickened, almost 5 minutes. Season with salt and dark pepper.

Squashed Potato Au Gratin
Somewhere, at some point, somebody planning an extraordinary event supper was solidified with uncertainty with respect to whether to serve squashed potatoes or potatoes au gratin. Both are classic sides that combine impeccably with any favor occasion

primary courses, so how to select? I cruel, you can't make both. Or can you?

Affirm, I'll concede to being that certain somebody battling with the choice. So I stacked them up and was able to have my pounded potatoes and potatoes au gratin as well.

Other than its marvelous appearance and being decently straightforward to create, the surface of the ultimate dish was very noteworthy. The squashed potatoes felt and tasted like mashed potatoes and, whereas the cut layer of potatoes on best wasn't as creamy as the classic form, it was everything you need in a potatoes au gratin formula and more.

So, whether it's for an occasion supper, or fair a few irregular weeknights, I truly do hope you donate this an attempt before long. Appreciate!

Ingredients

Pounded Potato Base:

6 expansive reddish brown potatoes, peeled and quartered

3 tablespoons legitimate salt

1/2 container cold unsalted butter, cut in pieces

salt to taste

1 squeeze cayenne

3/4 container drain

4 ounces Comte, Gruyere, or Cheddar cheese, destroyed

Au Gratin Potato Topping:

4 huge reddish brown potatoes, peeled and split

2 teaspoons legitimate salt

naturally ground dark pepper to taste

2 tablespoons softened butter

2 ounces Comte cheese, Gruyere cheese, or Cheddar cheese, destroyed

1/2 cup grated Parmigiano-Reggiano cheese

Headings

Preheat the stove to 450 degrees F (230 degrees C). Butter a 13x9-inch preparing dish.

For the crushed potato, incorporate quartered chestnut potatoes to a pot with 3 tablespoons salt and adequate water to cover by 2 inches. Bring to a bubble over tall warm; diminish warm to medium and stew until delicate when pierced with a sharp cut, but not falling apart, 15 to 20 minutes. Deplete exceptionally well.

Return potatoes to the pot, and pound until nearly smooth. Include butter, salt, and cayenne. Squash until smooth.

Include drain and the 4 ounces destroyed cheese, and squash and blend until equitably combined. Spread equitably into the arranged heating dish, and smooth the beat. Season the best with salt and crisply ground dark pepper.

For the au gratin potato layer, cut each half potato into 1/8-inch cuts.

Fan the potato out marginally at a point, and put on beat of pounded potatoes. Rehash with remaining potato parts to cover the surface, making 4 lines across by 2 potato parts long, utilizing 8 halves add up to. Depending on the estimate of potato and dish, you will ought to adjust the format to cover.

Generously salt cut potatoes, and brush liberally with softened butter. Scramble the 2 ounces destroyed cheese on best, and wrap up with ground Parmigiano-Reggiano.

Prepare within the preheated broiler until cut potatoes on top are delicate when penetrated with a cut, approximately 1 hour.

Yummy Sweet Potato Casserole
A conventional occasion table wouldn't be total without a sweet potato casserole. Superbly flavored and topped with an irresistible pecan topping, this is often the as it were sweet potato casserole formula you'll ever require.

How to Form Sweet Potato Casserole

You'll discover the total, step-by-step formula underneath — but here's a brief diagram of what you'll be able anticipate once you make this top-rated sweet potato casserole:

Cook and pound the sweet potatoes.

Blend the casserole fixings and exchange to a heating dish.

Make the topping and sprinkle it over the sweet potato blend.

Heat until the topping is gently browned.

Might You at any point Make Yam Dish Early?

Yes, you'll prepare this sweet potato casserole one to two days in advance. It's a great way to induce a head begin on Thanksgiving! To form ahead, basically get ready the filling and topping independently — but do not prepare anything however. Firmly cover the heating dish and put the topping in an airtight holder. Store them both in the fridge until you're prepared to cook.

On the big day, sprinkle the topping onto the filling and heat concurring to the headings (you will need to include a few minutes to the preparing time to account for the cold temperature).

How to Warm Sweet Potato Casserole

To warm this sweet potato casserole, cover with foil and heat in a stove preheated to 350 degrees F for 20-25 minutes (or until warmed through).

Can You Solidify Sweet Potato Casserole?

Yes, you'll solidify sweet potato casserole. Heat the filling concurring to the headings (ideally in a thwart heating skillet) without including the topping. Permit the casserole to cool, at that point wrap the whole heating dish firmly in thwart. Solidify for up to three months. Defrost within the fridge overnight. Add the topping and reheat in the stove concurring to the bearings above.

Fixings

Sweet Potatoes:

4 mugs peeled, cubed sweet potatoes

2 expansive eggs, beaten

½ glass white sugar

½ container drain

4 tablespoons butter, mellowed

½ teaspoon vanilla extricate

½ teaspoon salt

Pecan Topping:

½ glass stuffed brown sugar

⅓ container all-purpose flour

3 tablespoons butter, relaxed

½ container chopped pecans

Bearings

Preheat stove to 325 degrees F (165 degrees C).

Get ready sweet potatoes:

Put sweet potatoes in a medium pot and cover with water. Cook over medium-high warm until delicate, 10 to 15 minutes. Deplete and exchange to an expansive bowl.

Squash depleted sweet potatoes with a fork. Include eggs; blend until well combined. Include sugar, drain, butter, vanilla, and salt; blend until smooth. Exchange to a 9x13-inch preparing dish.

Make topping:

Blend brown sugar and flour together in a medium bowl. Cut in butter with a baked good cutter until blend is coarse and looks like peas; do not overmix. Blend in pecans. Sprinkle topping over sweet potato blend.

Heat within the preheated broiler until topping is softly browned, around 30 minutes.

Butter Flaky Pie Outside

In the event that you're scared by making hand crafted pie dough, you've come to the correct put. This flaky pie hull is culminating for apprentice bread cooks and prepared experts — it'll rapidly ended up a staple in your formula box.

Pie Hull Fixings

You'll require fair four fixings for this top-rated flaky pie outside formula:

Flour:

This flaky pie hull formula begins with all-purpose flour.

Salt:

A squeeze of salt improves the flavor and advances a delicate, wet hull.

Butter:

Cold butter includes wealthy flavor and makes steam because it softens, guaranteeing a flawlessly flaky wrapped up item.

Water:

Cold water acts as an authoritative operator which holds the dry fixings together. It too contributes to the flakiness of the hull because it dissipates.

What Makes a Pie Outside Flaky?

When it comes to making a flaky pie outside, it's all approximately the fat (in this case, butter). The fat works in two ways:

It coats the flour, anticipating it from retaining the fluid and making gluten. As well much gluten produces a thick, chewy hull.

As the fat dissolves amid baking, it clears out discuss pockets within the batter. The pockets fill with steam and grow, making layers of flaky cake hull.

For the flakiest outside, make beyond any doubt your fixings are as cold as conceivable to anticipate the fat from softening some time recently it makes it to the stove. It too makes a difference to work with cold hands and, in the event that conceivable, a marble rolling stick and cutting board.

How to Create a Flaky Pie Outside?

You'll discover the total, step-by-step recipe below — but here's a brief diagram of what you'll be able anticipate after you make this flaky pie hull:

Combine the flour and salt.

Cut within the cold butter until the blend takes after coarse scraps.

Include the cold water a tablespoon at a time.

Wrap the batter in plastic wrap and refrigerate for at slightest 4 hours or overnight.

Roll the mixture into a circle, at that point press it into a pie plate. Trim the abundance and woodwind the edges.

Fixings

1 ¼ mugs all-purpose flour

¼ teaspoon salt

½ glass butter, diced and then chilled

14 cup ice water, or as much as necessary

Headings

Accumulate all fixings.

Combine flour and salt in a huge bowl. Utilize a pale blender to cut in chilled, diced butter until blend takes after coarse pieces.

Include 1 tablespoon cold water at a time, blending with a spatula or your hands until the batter comes together; you may need less than 1/4 glass water.

Shape dough into a circle, wrap in plastic, and refrigerate for at slightest 4 hours or overnight.

Put chilled mixture on a liberally floured surface and roll out to an 11-inch circle, adding more flour to your rolling pin as required.

Carefully roll mixture onto the rolling stick, at that point unroll over a 9-inch pie dish. Press mixture equitably into the foot and sides of the dish. Trim any excess batter and woodwind the edges.

Blind-bake or fill and heat as coordinated in your pie formula

Stuffing Bread Pudding

Stuffing Bread Pudding Ingredients

These are the ingredients you'll ought to make this stuffing bread pudding formula:

Bread:

Begin with six mugs of delicate cubed bread.

Butter:

Cook the vegetables in dissolved butter.

Vegetables:

You'll require a yellow onion and celery.

Seasonings:

Season the stuffed bread pudding with new garlic, dried thyme, dried savvy, dried rosemary, salt, and pepper. White wine vinegar:

White wine vinegar includes welcome brightness and makes a difference deglaze the skillet.

Eggs:

Eggs keep the stuffing from drying out and offer assistance tie the fixings together.

Half-and-half:

Half-and-half loans moisture and wealthy flavor.

Cheese:

You'll require a combination of destroyed gouda and ground Parmesan cheeses.

How to Create Stuffing Bread Pudding?

You'll discover the complete, step-by-step recipe below — but here's a brief diagram of what you'll be able anticipate once you make homemade stuffing bread pudding:

Toast the bread 3d shapes.

Cook the vegetables in butter until the onions are translucent, at that point include the seasonings.

Include white wine vinegar and cook for 1 diminutive, mixing and scratching the dish.

Combine the toasted bread 3d shapes and onion blend in one bowl, at that point combine the eggs with the half-and-half and cheeses in another bowl.

Combine the bowls, at that point spread the blend in an arranged preparing dish.

Refrigerate for two hours or overnight, at that point let the blend come to room temperature.

Bake until the center is set and the beat is brilliant brown.

Fixings

6 glasses 3/4-inch cubes delicate sandwich bread

1/4 container unsalted butter

1 1/2 glasses chopped yellow onions (almost 1 1/2 onions)

1 glass chopped celery

3 clove cloves garlic

1 teaspoon dried thyme or 1 tablespoon chopped new thyme

1 teaspoon dried sage or 1 tablespoon chopped new sage

1 teaspoon dried rosemary or 1 tablespoon slashed new rosemary1 teaspoon salt

1 teaspoon crisply ground dark pepper

2 tablespoons white wine vinegar

1/4 cup chopped new parsley

4 expansive eggs

2 glasses half-and-half

1 glass destroyed Gouda cheese

3/4 glass naturally ground Parmesan cheese

Bearings

Assemble all fixings. Preheat grill to 350 degrees F (175 degrees C). Oil a 2-quart preparing dish; set aside.

Spread bread on a huge preparing sheet. Ake until delicately brilliant and toasted, approximately 20 minutes, mixing once midway through. Turn stove off.

Liquefy butter in an expansive skillet over medium warm. Include onions and celery, cook blending regularly, until translucent, approximately 5 minutes.

Include garlic, thyme, sage, rosemary, salt and pepper. Proceed to cook and blend until garlic is fragrant, almost 2 minutes. Include white wine vinegar and cook, blending, until generally dissipated, 1 diminutive.

Combine toasted bread 3d shapes, onion blend, and parsley in a huge bowl; set aside.

Combine eggs, half-and-half, gouda, and Parmesan in a medium bowl. Include to bread 3d shape blend, blend to combine.

Spread bread blend equitably within the arranged heating dish. Cover and refrigerate 2 hours to overnight. Let bread pudding stand at room temperature for 20 minutes some time recently preparing. Preheat oven to 350 degrees F (175 degrees C)

Prepare until center of bread pudding is set, beat is brilliant brown and a cut embedded within the center comes out clean (160 degrees F or 71 degrees C inside temperature), around 45 minutes. Let stand 10 minutes some time as of late serving.

A Basically Culminate Cook Turkey

Nothing shouts "Thanksgiving" very like a pleasant broil turkey commendable of a Norman Rockwell portray. Accept it or not, an inconceivably dazzling occasion table of your dreams is inside reach — learn precisely how to cook a turkey with this simple formula.

Broil Turkey Ingredients

You would like fair five fixings to create this top-rated cook turkey formula:

Turkey:

This formula calls for an 18-pound entirety turkey.

Stuffing:

You'll require eight glasses of arranged stuffing. Utilize store-bought or attempt one of our best formulas for hand crafted stuffing.

Butter:

Salted butter, rubbed onto the skin, guarantees a delicious cook turkey each time.

Salt and pepper:

This broil turkey is basically prepared with fair salt and pepper. Of course, you'll include more flavors to suit your taste.

Turkey stock:

The winged creature is cooked in and seasoned with store-bought or hand crafted turkey stock.

How to Broil a Turkey?

You'll discover the total, step-by-step formula below — but here's what you'll anticipate once you make this top-rated broil turkey:

Plan the turkey:

Expel the turkey neck and giblets. Pat the turkey dry with paper towels, at that point put it (breast-side up) on a rack in a simmering container.

Stuff and season the turkey:

Fill the cavity with stuffing. Rub the skin with butter, at that point season with salt and pepper. Pour two glasses of stock into the broiling dish and freely tent the turkey with thwart.

Cook the turkey:

Cook, seasoning with stock each 30 minutes, for around two and half hours. Include more stock as the drippings dissipate. Expel the thwart and proceed broiling until a meat thermometer embedded into the thickest portion of the thigh peruses 165 degrees F.

How Long to Broil a Turkey?

The 18-pound turkey is simmered for almost four hours at 325 degrees F. On the off chance that your turkey is bigger or littler than 18 pounds, you'll have to be alter the cooking time. Learn more in our Turkey Cooking Time Direct.

Do You Would like a Roaster?

Nope! Whereas an electric roaster is certainly decent to have, this formula was created for the stove.

Fixings

1 (18 pound) entirety turkey

8 glasses arranged stuffing

½ glass unsalted butter, relaxed

salt and naturally ground dark pepper to taste

1 ½ quarts turkey stock, partitioned

Directions

Accumulate all ingredients. Set the stove to 325 degrees Fahrenheit (165 degrees Celsius). Put a rack within the most reduced position of the stove.

Evacuate turkey neck and giblets. Flush turkey and pat dry with paper towels, and put breast-side up, on a rack in a simmering skillet.

Freely fill turkey depth with stuffing. Rub skin with butter, at that point season with salt and pepper.

Pour 2 mugs of turkey stock into the broiling container.

Freely tent turkey with aluminum thwart, and broil turkey for 2 1/2 hours, basting with skillet juices each 30 minutes. When drippings dissipate, include remaining stock to the container, 1 to 2 glasses at a time.

Remove thwart and proceed broiling until a meat thermometer inserted in thickest part of thigh peruses 165 degrees F (75 degrees C), approximately 1 1/2 hours more.

Exchange turkey to a huge serving platter. Let stand for 20 to 30 minutes some time recently carving.

Sweet Potato Dump Cake

This sweet potato dump cake formula, created in our test kitchen by culinary master Kathryn Standing, is perfect for all your holiday potluck needs.

Sweet Potato Dump Cake Ingredients

These are the fixings you'll have to be make this simple sweet potato dump cake formula:

Canned sweet potatoes:

This formula begins with two cans of sweet potatoes in light syrup, depleted.

Butter:

You'll require two sticks of salted butter, partitioned.

Sweetened condensed drain:

Sweetened condensed drain is the wanton mystery fixing.

Vanilla:

Take the flavor up a score with vanilla extricate.

Flavors:

Pumpkin pie zest includes hot, warm, cozy flavor. Use store-bought pumpkin pie zest or make you possess blend at home.

Cake blend:

Utilize store-bought boxed yellow cake mix or boxed spice cake blend.

Pecans:

Chopped pecans are discretionary, but they include welcome crunch and flavor.

How to Form Sweet Potato Dump Cake

The complete, step-by-step recipe is provided below; however, here is a brief description of what to expect when making handcrafted sweet potato dump cake:

Beat the sweet potatoes, an adhere of liquefied butter, sweetened condensed drain, vanilla, and zest in an expansive blending bowl until nearly smooth.

Spread the sweet potato blend equitably into the arranged dish, at that point sprinkle with cake blend.

Put cold butter pieces equally over cake blend and sprinkle with pecans.

Prepare until brilliant brown and set.

Ingredients

2 (15 ounce) cans sweet potatoes in light syrup, depleted

1/2 container salted butter, melted

1 (14-ounce) can sweetened condensed drain

1 tablespoon vanilla extricate

1 tablespoon pumpkin pie flavor

1 bundle (2 layer) spice cake mix or yellow cake blend

1/2 cup salted butter, cold, cut into little pieces

1/2 container chopped pecans (discretionary)

whipped cream or vanilla ice cream, to serve, if wanted

Bearings

Assemble fixings. Preheat the stove to 350 degrees F (180 degrees C). Oil a 9x13-inch heating dish; set aside.

Combine depleted sweet potatoes, 1/2 container dissolved butter, sweetened condensed drain, vanilla, and pumpkin pie flavor in an expansive bowl. Beat until nearly smooth with an electric blender. There may still be a few little chunks of sweet potato.

Spread sweet potato blend equitably into the arranged container. Sprinkle cake blend over the sweet potato blend. Put cold butter pieces equitably over cake blend. Sprinkle with pecans, on the off chance that utilizing.

Prepare until brilliant brown and set, approximately 45 minutes. Cool at slightest 20 minutes in container some time recently serving. Serve with whipped cream or ice cream, in the event that craved.

How to Form Apple Pie?

You'll discover a nitty gritty ingredient list and step-by-step enlightening within the formula underneath, but let's go over the essentials:

Apple Pie Ingredients

These are the straightforward fixings to create this top-rated apple pie formula:

Apples:

This formula calls for eight little Granny Smith apples.

Butter and flour:

The filling begins with butter and all-purpose flour cooked into a glue.

Sugars:

A mix of white and brown sugar makes the culminate sweet flavor with an imply of warmth.

Pie outside:

Utilize a store-bought twofold hull pie baked good or make you possess at domestic.

Best Apples for Apple Pie

This formula calls for Granny Smith apples for some reasons:

Their solidness implies they will hold their shape amid cooking and their tart flavor flawlessly equalizations out the sweetness of the sugar. A few bread cooks lean toward utilizing Granny Smith apples in combination with a somewhat sweeter variety, such as Honeycrisp.

How to Form an Apple Pie?

Here's an exceptionally brief diagram of what you'll anticipate once you make this old-fashioned apple pie at home:

Make the filling:

On the stove, make a glue with flour and butter. Include the sugar and water and bring to a bubble. Stew, at that point evacuate from warm.

Collect the pie:

Press one hull into a pie plate. Put the cut apples on the foot hull. Utilize the best outside to form a grid hull agreeing to the formula underneath. Pour the butter-sugar blend over the cross section hull.

Heat the pie:

Prepare the pie in a preheated stove until the apples are delicate and the outside is brilliant brown.

How Long to Heat Apple Pie?

You'll warm the pie at 425 degrees F for 15 minutes, by then you'll lessen the temperature to 350 degrees F and continue planning for 35-

45 minutes. All in all, the pie will prepare for almost one hour, give or take a couple of minutes. You'll know the pie is done when the apples are delicate and the crust may be a beautiful brilliant brown color.

Does Apple Pie Require to Be Refrigerated?

Cover the cooled pie firmly with thwart and store at room temperature for up to two days or within the fridge for up to four days.

Can You Solidify Apple Pie?

Yes! Since this apple pie doesn't contain custard or cream, it'll solidify very pleasantly. Wrap the pie in two layers of plastic wrap and one layer of aluminum thwart. Put it in an airtight holder or cover in another layer of thwart. Crush out the abundance discuss and solidify for up to three months.

Fixings

8 little Granny Smith apples, or as required

½ glass unsalted butter

3 tablespoons all-purpose flour

½ container white sugar

½ container pressed brown sugar

¼ glass water

1 (9 inch) double-crust pie baked good, defrosted

Headings

Peel and center apples, at that point meagerly cut. Set aside.

Preheat the stove to 425 degrees F (220 degrees C)

Liquefy butter in a saucepan over medium heat. Add flour and mix to form a glue; cook until fragrant, around 1 to 2 minutes. Include both sugars and water; bring to a bubble. Diminish the warm to moo and stew for 3 to 5 minutes. Evacuate from the warm.

Press one baked good into the foot and up the sides of a 9-inch pie dish. Roll out remaining pastry so it'll overhang the pie by approximately 1/2 inch. Cut pastry into eight 1-inch strips.

Put cut apples into the foot hull, shaping a slight hill. Lay four cake strips vertically and equally divided over apples, using longer strips within the center and shorter strips at the edges.

Make a grid hull:

Overlay the primary and third strips all the way back so they're nearly falling off the pie. Lay one of the unused strips oppositely over the moment and fourth strips, at that point unfurl the primary and third strips back into their unique position.

Crease the second and fourth vertical strips back. Lay one of the three unused strips oppositely over top. Unfurl the second and fourth strips back into their original position.

Rehash Steps 6 and 7 to weave within the final two strips of cake. Fold and trim abundance batter at the edges as vital, and squeeze to secure.

Gradually and delicately pour sugar-butter blend over cross section hull, making beyond any doubt it leaks over cut apples. Brush a few onto cross section, but make beyond any doubt it doesn't run off the sides.

Bake in the preheated stove for 15 minutes. Decrease the temperature to 350 degrees F (175 degrees C) and proceed preparing until apples are delicate, 35 to 45 minutes.

New Cranberry Sauce
The leading things in life are regularly the best — and this new cranberry sauce, made with fair three fixings, is confirmation.

How to Form New Cranberry Sauce

It couldn't be simpler to make this new cranberry sauce with fair three ingredients. You'll discover the complete, step-by-step formula underneath — but here's a brief outline of what you'll expect:

Bring the water to a boil, at that point blend within the sugar and cook until it is broken up. Include the cranberries and bring to a bubble once more. Diminish the warm and continue cooking until the berries have popped and the sauce is chunky. Exchange the sauce to a serving dish or jars to cool totally. Blend with a fork some time recently serving.

Fixings

1 container water

1 glass white sugar

1 (12 ounce) bundle new cranberries (such as Sea Spray

Headings

Assemble all fixings.

Bring water to a bubble in a pot; include sugar and cook until sugar is broken down, approximately 5 minutes.

Mix cranberries into the pot and bring to a bubble. Decrease warm to moo, and stew until cranberries have popped and sauce is chunky, around 10 minutes or longer for craved consistency. The longer you cook it, the less chunky it'll be.

Pour sauce into a serving dish or containers and cover until prepared to use; the pectin within the cranberries will make the cranberry sauce gel because it cools.

Blend cranberry sauce with a fork some time recently serving

Speedy Brussels and Bacon

Fixings

6 cuts bacon

½ tablespoon olive oil

3 shallots, chopped

1 (16 ounce) bundle solidified Brussels grows, defrosted and divided

Bearings

Cook the bacon in an expansive skillet over medium-high warm until fresh; deplete on paper towels and disintegrate.

Warm the olive oil in an expansive skillet over medium-high warm. Cook and mix the onion within the oil until delicate; blend within the bacon and cook until bacon is warmed through. Include the Brussels grows; cook and mix until the grows are browned, 7 to 10 minutes.

Butternut Squash Cheesecake
This butternut squash cheesecake is genius—it's lighter, more flavorful, and just as wealthy and wanton as its pumpkin cheesecake cousin. This one is heated Basque cheesecake-style, hot and quick, needs no crust, and will be pleasantly browned on best. It may split, but

truly, do we care when it is this rich and delightful?

Fixings

1 huge butternut squash, simmered to abdicate

1 1/2 glasses pounded squash

16 ounces' cream cheese, mollified

3/4 container white sugar

1/4 container all-purpose flour

1 teaspoon legitimate salt

1/4 glass maple syrup

1/2 teaspoon ground cinnamon

1/2 teaspoon ground ginger

1/4 teaspoon naturally ground nutmeg

1 1/2 teaspoons vanilla extricate

5 huge eggs

1 container overwhelming cream

Headings

Preheat the broiler to 400 degrees F (200 degrees C). Oil a 10-inch spring form container, line with material, and set aside. Line a heating sheet with material.

Cut butternut squash into thick crosswise cuts, expel seeds, and put on the lined preparing sheet.

Broil within the preheated broiler until exceptionally delicate, almost 1 hour. When cool sufficient to handle, isolated the substance from the skin; discard skin. Squash squash until smooth, measure out 1 1/2 glasses, and set aside to cool totally. Save any remaining squash for another utilize.

Increment the stove temperature to 425 degrees F (220 degrees C).

Include mellowed cream cheese, sugar, flour, and salt to a bowl, and cream beside a spatula until exceptionally smooth.

Include maple syrup, 1 1/2 glasses mashed butternut squash, cinnamon, ginger, and nutmeg. Blend with an electric blender or whisk until combined; blend in vanilla. Incorporate eggs, each in turn, beating great after every extension Mix in cream.

Pour hitter into arranged spring form container. Tap the dish delicately on the counter to settle the hitter.

Prepare within the preheated stove until cheesecake is nearly completely set, 50 to 60 minutes. The center ought to squirm exceptionally marginally in the event that the container is shaken back and forward. On the off chance that the center appears soupy, proceed heating for some more minutes.

Remove and let cool for 5 minutes. Run a lean cut between the exterior edge of the cheesecake and the interior of the spring form ring to discharge cheesecake from the ring; it will contract because it cools. Let cool 30 minutes more, then expel exterior ring.

Refrigerate cheesecake for a number of hours or up to overnight some time recently serving.

Bacon-Garlic Green Beans
This family-favorite vegetable side dish of green beans is straightforward and fast to make. Awesome for family meals, Thanksgiving, or any event. You'll substitute lime zest for the lemon get-up-and-go in case craved.

Fixings

3 pounds' new green beans, trimmed

4 cuts bacon

1 glass butter

4 cloves garlic, minced

½ teaspoon lemon get-up-and-go

Bearings

Put green beans in a pot and cover with water; bring to a bubble. Diminish warm to medium-low and stew until beans begin to mellow, around 10 minutes. Deplete water, clearing out beans within the pot.

Put bacon strips on a microwave-safe plate and cook within the microwave until crisp, around 2 minutes. Cool and disintegrate bacon.

Mix butter and bacon into beans within the pot and return to medium heat; cook and stir until butter dissolves, 2 to 3 minutes. Include garlic; cook and mix until fragrant, 3 to 4 minutes. Best with lemon get-up-and-go and mix.

Cook's Notes:

Expel the bacon for a healthier dish. Be that as it may, including the bacon could be a great option that includes flavor to the beans.

Sodden and Savory Stuffing

There's nothing better at the occasions than a huge bowl of classic Thanksgiving stuffing:

the feathery surface and savory flavors like rosemary, parsley, and thyme can make anybody feel warm and cozy. We overhauled this classic recipe with the wealthy flavor of Swanson® Chicken Broth, but it's too a incredible establishment that you simply can customize with your family's favorite add-ins to total your Thanksgiving supper.

Fixings

¼ glass butter

1 container coarsely chopped celery

1 glass coarsely chopped onion

2 ½ glasses Swanson® Chicken Broth

1 (12 ounce) bundle Pepperidge Farm® Herb Prepared Stuffing

Bearings

Warm the broiler to 350 degrees F (175 degrees C).

Warm the butter in a 3-quart pan over medium warm. Include the celery and onion and cook for 5 minutes or until tender-crisp, mixing every so often.

Include Swanson® Chicken Broth to the pan and warm to a bubble. Expel the pan from the warm. Include the stuffing and blend gently. Spoon the stuffing blend into a lubed 9x13x2-inch heating dish. Cover the heating dish.

Prepare for 30 minutes or until the stuffing blend is hot.

Cranberry & Pecan Stuffing

Mix 1/2 glass each dried cranberries and chopped pecans into the stuffing blend some time recently heating.

Wiener & Mushroom Stuffing

Include 1 container cut mushrooms to the vegetables amid cooking. Mix 1/2-pound pork frankfurter, cooked and disintegrated, into the stuffing blend some time recently heating.

Make Ahead:

Plan as coordinated but don't heat Cover and refrigerate for as long as 24 hours. To heat, warm the stove to 350 degrees F (175 degrees C). Prepare, revealed, for 30 minutes or until hot.

Great and Simple Velvety Corn Casserole

This corn casserole is really the foremost delightful stuff! A bit like a cross between corn soufflé and a somewhat sweet corn pudding. Attempt it! I know you'll adore how simple it is to plan, but you'll particularly adore the taste!

This corn casserole will be a welcome expansion to any table. Whether you're cooking for an extraordinary event or a normal weeknight, this creamy corn casserole formula will unquestionably get to be a staple in your revolution.

How to Create Corn Casserole?

You'll discover a point by point fixing list and step-by-step informational within the recipe underneath, but let's go over the essentials:

Corn Casserole Fixings

These are the easy-to-find fixings you'll have to be make this top-rated velvety corn casserole formula

Canned corn:

You'll require one can of entire part corn and one can of creamed corn.

Cornbread blend:

A bundle of dry cornbread blend is the mystery fixing in this alternate route creamed corn formula.

Acrid cream:

Acrid cream loans creaminess and an imply of tang.

Butter:

Softened butter includes abundance and flavor.

Eggs:

Two eggs donate the casserole dampness and tie the fixings together.

How Do You Make Corn Casserole?

It couldn't be simpler to create this custom made corn casserole:

Essentially blend the fixings until they're well-combined, exchange to a preparing dish, and heat until a toothpick embedded into the center comes out clean.

Can You Make Corn Casserole Ahead of Time?

Yes! You'll make corn casserole up to two days in advance. Cover the cooled casserole firmly with capacity wrap and store in the fridge. Warm in a broiler preheated to 300 degrees F for 10-20 minutes (or until warmed through).

Can You Solidify Corn Casserole?

Yes, you'll be able solidify corn casserole for up to three months. Wrap the casserole in a layer of capacity wrap, at that point in a layer of aluminum thwart. Thaw within the fridge, at that point warm within the broiler or microwave.

Fixings

1 (15 ounce) can entirety kernel corn, depleted

1 (14.75 ounce) can creamed corn

1 (8.5 ounce) bundle dry cornbread blend

1 cup acrid cream

½ cup butter, softened

2 expansive eggs, beaten

Bearings

Preheat the oven to 350 degrees F (175 degrees C) Softly oil a 9x9-inch heating dish.

Blend entire and creamed corn, cornbread blend, acrid cream, softened butter, and eggs together in a medium bowl until well combined. Spoon blend into the arranged dish.

Heat in the preheated broiler until the best is brilliant brown and a toothpick embedded in the center comes out clean, approximately 45 minutes.

Turkey Brine

This can be a delicious turkey brine formula for any poultry. It'll make your bird very juicy, and sauce to pass on for! Usually sufficient brine for a 10- to 18- pound turkey.

A good brine is the key to a succulent, flavor, and delicate turkey that will impress everyone at your table. Searching for the finest turkey brine formula? We've got you secured.

This top-rated damp brine, prepared with fragrant fixings like rosemary and thyme, will gotten to be an annual tradition in your house.

What Is Brining?

Brine includes dampness and flavor to all sorts of meats, counting turkey. Since turkey is an incline meat without a part of fat, this step guarantees your supper isn't extreme and dry.

At its least difficult, a brine could be an essential arrangement of water and salt. Numerous brine formulas, in spite of the fact that, contain additional flavors and seasonings to ramp up the flavor.

**Damp vs. Dry Brine
There are two types of brines:**

damp and dry. A damp brine (such as this one) immerses the turkey in salt water. The meat assimilates the water and the salt makes a difference the muscles hold the fluid, which comes about in a delicious turkey that isn't overflowing water.

A dry brine, in the interim, doesn't contain fluid. It works because the salt blends with the meat juices and is ingested into the turkey.

Turkey Brine Ingredients

This brine is simple to throw together with fixings you likely as of now have on hand. Here's what you'll require:

Vegetable Broth:

You can utilize store-bought or hand crafted vegetable broth as the base for this formula. Chicken broth will moreover work on the off chance that that's what you have on hand.

Salt:

Sea salt infuses the feathered creature with savory flavor through osmosis. It moreover makes a difference keep the meat delicate and delicious.

Rosemary, Sage, Thyme, and Savory:

Natural herbs and spices like rosemary, sage, thyme, and savory (a fragrant herb within the mint family) include flavor and complexity.

Water:

Ice water includes volume to the brine. Also, it keeps the turkey succulent and tender.

How to Create Turkey Brine?

Making the brine couldn't be simpler:

Just combine all the fixings (other than the ice water) on the stove and bring to a boil. Blend the blend habitually. When the salt is broken up, evacuate from warm and let the brine cool totally.

How to Brine a Turkey?

There are a couple of distinctive ways to brine a turkey. For this method, you'll fair ought to follow a number of simple steps. You'll discover the complete recipe below, but here's a brief overview of what you'll be able anticipate:

Make the brine by bubbling the primary six fixings in a stockpot.

Let the brine cool slightly, at that point exchange it to a bucket or stockpot. Add the ice water and **stir.**

Put the prepared turkey within the brine and refrigerate overnight.

When your turkey is done brining, expel it from the bucket and deplete carefully.

Dispose of the brine, making sure to purify anything it comes in contact with.

Cook the turkey utilizing the strategy of your choosing.

Fixings

1-gallon vegetable broth

1 container ocean salt

1 tablespoon pulverized dried rosemary

1 tablespoon dried sage

1 tablespoon dried thyme

1 tablespoon dried savory

1-gallon ice water

Headings

Assemble all fixings.

Combine vegetable broth, ocean salt, rosemary, sage, thyme, and savory in a huge stockpot. Bring to a bubble, mixing as often as possible to be beyond any doubt salt is broken up. Evacuate from warm, and let cool to room temperature.

When the broth blend is cool, pour it into a clean 5-gallon bucket. Mix within the ice water.

Wash and dry your turkey. Make beyond any doubt you've got expelled the innards. Put the turkey, breast down, into the brine. Make sure that the depression gets filled. Put the bucket within the fridge for 8 hours, or overnight

Evacuate the turkey carefully, depleting off the abundance brine and pat dry. Dispose of overabundance brine.

Cook the turkey as desired saving the drippings for sauce. Be beyond any doubt that brined turkeys cook 20 to 30 minutes speedier so observe the temperature gage.

**Fiery chicken & avocado wraps
Strategy**

STEP

Blend the chicken with the lime juice, chilli powder and garlic.

STEP

Warm the oil in a non-stick searing container at that point broil the chicken for one or two of mins – it'll cook exceptionally rapidly so keep an eye on it. Meanwhile, warm the wraps taking after the pack informational or, in case you've got a gas hob, warm them over the fire to marginally char them. Don't let them dry out or they are troublesome to roll.

STEP

Squash half an avocado onto each wrap, include the peppers to the container to warm them through at that point pile onto the wraps with the chicken, and sprinkle over the coriander. Roll up, cut in half and eat together with your fingers.

Fixings

1 chicken breast (approx 180g), daintily cut at a point

liberal press juice 0.5 lime

½ tsp mellow chilli powder

1 garlic clove, chopped

1 tsp olive oil

2 seeded wraps

1 avocado, split and stoned

1 simmered ruddy pepper from a jolt, cut

a number of sprigs coriander, chopped

**Firm destroyed chicken
Strategy**

STEP

Cut the chicken into lean strips. Pour over 2 tbsp of the soy and marinate within the fridge, covered, for 1 hr.

STEP

In the meantime, warm 1 tbsp of the oil in a wok or deep frying skillet over a medium warm and cook the peppers for 3-4 mins until just starting to relax. Evacuate with an opened spoon and set aside.

STEP 3

Spread the cornflour out in a shallow bowl. Season, at that point include the marinated chicken strips and hurl to coat well.

STEP 4

Fill a wok or profound searing dish with the oil so it's about ½cm profound, at that point warm to medium-high. Carefully include the chicken in bunches, cooking for 3-4 mins, utilizing tongs to turn routinely until brilliant and fresh. Expel with an opened spoon and put on a plate lined with kitchen paper to deplete.

STEP 5

Blend together the remaining soy, sweet chilli, garlic glue and sesame oil in a huge bowl. Include the cooked peppers, firm chicken and toss together until coated all over and sticky. Serve sprinkled with the spring onions.

Fixings

320g pack chicken scaled down breast filets

2½ tbsp light soy sauce

vegetable oil, for singing

1 red pepper, deseeded and daintily cut

1 green pepper, deseeded and daintily cut

3 tbsp cornflour

3 tbsp sweet chilli sauce

1 tbsp garlic and ginger glue

1 tbsp sesame oil

2 spring onions, trimmed and finely cut

Solid hamburger chow mein

Strategy

STEP

Cook the noodles taking after pack enlightening. In the meantime, warm half the oil in a wok and stir-fry the meat over a tall warm for 30 seconds until browned. Tip onto a plate, set aside, at that point include the remaining oil to the wok. Stir-fry the onion and ginger until relaxed. Include a drop of water to avoid burning, in case required and cook secured for 2-3 mins.

STEP

Blend within the mushrooms and garlic, and broil until they begin to relax (around 3 mins), at that point include the beansprouts and cook for a miniature or two more until channeling hot.

STEP 3

Blend the tamari and vinegar together in a little bowl with 2 tbsp water. Include the depleted noodles to the wok, hurl well, then add the tamari blend, spring onions and the beef. Heat through in a few minutes of stir-frying. Season with bounty of dark pepper and serve.

Fixings

2 whole meal noodle nests (85g)

2 tsp rapeseed or sesame oil

200g incline filet steak, fat evacuated and cut into strips

1 little ruddy onion (100g), finely chopped

15g piece of ginger, peeled and finely chopped

160g chestnut mushrooms, thickly cut

2 garlic cloves, finely chopped

160g ready-to-eat beansprouts

1½ tsp tamari

1 tbsp brown rice vinegar

4 spring onions (65g), cut into inclining lengths

**Panuozzo sandwich
Strategy**

STEP 1

Put the flour in a huge bowl, at that point blend within the yeast and a huge squeeze of salt. Make a well within the middle, pour in 175ml warm water and the oil and bring in conjunction with a wooden spoon to make a soft, decently damp batter. Turn out onto a softly floured surface and work for 5-8 mins until smooth. Isolate the batter into four balls and organize on a floured plate, well dispersed apart. Cover with a tea towel and set aside for almost 40 mins-1 hr until multiplied in measure.

STEP 2

Warm the broiler to 240C/220C fan/gas 8 and put a heating tray in the stove to warm up. Roll the batter balls out on a floured surface into long baguette sticks around 22-25cm long, put on the hot plate and prepare for 10-12 mins until puffed up and brilliant, at that point take off to cool. Can be made a couple of hours ahead of heating.

STEP 3

To amass, part the bread down one side and perfectly layer in the tomato, ham, mozzarella and rocket, in case utilizing. Blend the pesto with the olive oil, sprinkle over, split and serve.

Fixings

For the batter

300g strong white bread flour, additionally additional for tidying

3g (approximately half a sachet) fast-action dried yeast

1 tbsp olive oil

For the filling

1 tomato, divided and sliced

4 cups cooked ham

150g mozzarella ball, cut and prepared

little modest bunch of rocket (discretionary)

6 tbsp pesto (see underneath for the formula)

1 tbsp olive oil

Kale caesar serving of mixed greens

Method

STEP 1

Combine the kale with 1 tbsp of the olive oil and a great squeeze of salt in an expansive bowl, and massage the oil into the clears out for a miniature some time recently setting aside to tenderise a little.

STEP 2

Warm the broiler to 200C/180C fan/gas 6. Diffuse the bread on an expansive simmering plate, at that point sprinkle over the remaining 1 tbsp oil. Hurl to coat the bread, at that point prepare for 10 mins until brilliant and fresh. Evacuate from the broiler and set aside.

STEP 3

Hurl together the kale, lettuce, avocado, in case utilizing, and shaved parmesan until equitably blended.

STEP 4

Combine the dressing fixings in a little bowl and blend together until well combined. You'll be able to do this in a jolt – put the top on and shake well. Extricate with a small water (it ought to be the consistency of yogurt), at that point pour over the serving of mixed greens. Scramble over the sourdough bread garnishes and hurl once more, at that point pound over a few dark pepper and serve.

Fixings

400g kale, extreme stems expelled and clears out torn into huge pieces

2 tbsp olive oil

2 thick cuts sourdough, torn into chunks

2 Small Diamond lettuces, clears out isolated

1 avocado, generally chopped (discretionary)

30g parmesan, shaved

For the dressing

1 garlic clove, finely ground

2 anchovies in oil, finely chopped

15g parmesan, finely ground

5 tbsp mayonnaise

1 tbsp white wine vinegar

Reuben sandwich

Strategy

STEP 1

Blend all the fixings for the mayonnaise, but the lemon juice, together in a bowl. Season to taste with the lemon squeeze, salt, and pepper.

STEP 2

Warm the flame broil to tall. Line a heating plate with heating material and organize the corned hamburger into four heaps on it, at that point beat with the cheese and barbecue until liquefied and bubbling.

STEP 3

Butter both sides of all the bread cuts. Warm a searing skillet over a medium warm and toast the bread cuts on both sides until brilliant.

Liberally spread the mayonnaise over one side of each bread cut. Beat four of the cuts, mayonnaise-side up, with the cheese-topped corned meat and the sauerkraut, at that point sandwich with the remaining bread cuts, mayonnaise-side down. Secure with cocktail sticks, at that point cut in half to serve.

Fixings

8 cuts corned meat

100g gruyère, cut

4 tbsp butter, mellowed

8 thick cuts rye bread

75g white sauerkraut

For the mayonnaise

100g mayonnaise

2 tbsp soured cream

1 little shallot, finely chopped

2 tbsp parsley, finely chopped

2 tbsp salted cucumber savor

½ tbsp creamed horseradish

½ tbsp Worcestershire sauce

2 dashes hot sauce

½ lemon, juiced

**Bulgur & quinoa lunch bowls
Strategy**

STEP 1

Tip the onion and bulgur blend into a dish, pour over 600ml water and mix in the thyme and bouillon. Cook, secured, over a moo warm for 15 mins, at that point take off to stand for 10 mins. All the fluid ought to presently be retained. When cool, evacuate the thyme and separate the bulgur between four bowls or plastic holders.

STEP 2

For the avocado topping, hurl all the fixings together but for the rocket. Heap onto two parcels of the bulgur and best with the rocket.

STEP 3

For the beetroot topping, to begin with heap the chickpeas on best, at that point hurl the beetroot with the tomato, mint, cumin, a great squeeze of cinnamon, the oil and vinegar. Hurl well, include the orange, at that point heap onto the remaining parcels of bulghur, scramble with the pine nuts and sprinkle with additional cinnamon. Chill within the cooler until required.

Fixings

For the bulgur base

1 huge onion, exceptionally finely chopped

150g bulgur and quinoa (this comes arranged mixed)2sprigs of thyme

2 tsp vegetable bouillon powder

For the avocado topping

1 avocado, split, destoned and chopped

2 tomatoes, cut into wedges

4 tbsp chopped basil

6 Kalamata olives, split

2 tsp additional virgin olive oil

2 tsp cider vinegar

2 enormous modest bunches of rocket

For the beetroot topping

210g can chickpeas, depleted

160g cooked beetroot, diced

2 tomatoes, cut into wedges

2 tbsp chopped mint

1 tsp cumin seeds

a few squeezes of ground cinnamon

2 tsp additional virgin olive oil

2 tsp cider vinegar

1 orange, cut into fragments

2 tbsp toasted pine nuts

Extreme chorizo ciabatta
Strategy

STEP 1

Warm broiler to 180C/160C fan/gas 4 and put the ciabatta in to warm up. Put a griddle container over a medium warm and cook the chorizo for 5 mins each side or until charred and cooked through.

STEP 2

Open up the warmed ciabatta and spread the pesto on the foot. Layer with the ruddy peppers, at that point the warm chorizo. Diffuse over the rocket, sandwich the ciabatta together, cut in two and serve.

Our Most Well-known Elective

Extreme crème burley

Goes well with

A star rating of 4.5 out of 5.

11 appraisals

A star rating of 4.6 out of 5.

86 evaluations

a rating of four stars out of five

9 appraisals

Supported substance

Comments, questions and tips

Rate this formula

What is your star rating out of 5?1 star out of 5

2 stars out of 5

3 stars out of 5

4 stars out of 5

5 stars out of 5

Select the sort of message you'd like to post

Select the sort of message you'd like to post

Comment

Address

Tip

Generally rating

A star rating of 4.5 out of 5.

15 appraisals

Be the primary to comment

We'd love to listen how you got on with this formula. Did you like it? Do you have got recommendations for conceivable swaps and increases? Or basically inquire us your questions...

Fixings

2 little or 1 expansive ciabatta

150g pack cooking chorizo, split lengthways

75g pesto

200g broiled ruddy peppers from a bump

modest bunch rocket

Chicken kiev quesadilla

Rosie Birkett

Strategy

STEP 1

Warm a non-stick singing skillet over a medium-high warm. Spread half the wrap with

2 tbsp delicate cheese and put within the container. Cover the other half with the cheddar, at that point beat with the spring onion, lemon pizzazz, parsley and chicken. Diffuse over the panko and speck the remaining delicate cheese over.

STEP 2

Crease the soft-cheese-spread side of the wrap over to shut the quesadilla. Cook for 3-4 mins until the cheese has liquefied and the best of the quesadilla is warm, so you know the chicken is warmed through. Cut and serve.

Fixings

1 expansive wrap or wheat tortilla

4 tbsp garlic and herb delicate cheese

50g cheddar, ground

1 spring onion, cut in half at that point cut lengthways into thick strips

½ lemon, zested

½ little pack flat-leaf parsley, chopped

100g cooked chicken thigh meat, cleaved into scaled down pieces

1 tbsp panko breadcrumbs

Egg & rocket pizzas
Sara Buenfeld

Strategy

STEP 1

Warm stove to 200C/180C fan/gas 6. Lay the tortillas on two preparing sheets, brush sparingly with the oil at that point heat for 3 mins. In the meantime, chop the pepper and tomatoes and blend with the tomato purée, flavoring and herbs. Turn the tortillas over and spread with the tomato blend, clearing out the middle free from any huge pieces of pepper or tomato.

STEP 2

Break an egg into the middle at that point return to the broiler for 10 mins or until the egg is fair set and the tortilla is firm circular the edges. Serve dispersed with the rocket and onion.

Fixings

2 seeded wraps

a small olive oil, for brushing

1 broiled ruddy pepper, from a jolt

2 tomatoes

2 tbsp tomato purée

1 tbsp chopped dill

2 tbsp chopped parsley

2 eggs

65g pack rocket

½ ruddy onion, exceptionally meagerly cut

Broccoli pasta serving of mixed greens with eggs & sunflower seeds

Strategy

STEP 1

Hard-boil the eggs for 8 mins, at that point shell and divide. In the interim, bubble the pasta for 5 mins, include the broccoli and beans, and cook 5 mins more or until everything is delicate.

STEP 2

Deplete, saving the water, at that point tip the pasta and veg into a bowl and mix within the miso, ginger, oil and 4 tbsp pasta water. Serve topped with the eggs and seeds.

Fixings

2 huge eggs

75g whole-wheat penne

160g broccoli florets

160g fine beans, trimmed and divided

1 tbsp white miso glue

1 tsp ground ginger

1 tbsp rapeseed oil

2 tbsp sunflower seeds

**Lime pickle rarebit
Strategy**

STEP 1

Liquefy the butter in a pan over a medium heat. Once frothing, tip within the flour and mustard powder and blend until a glue shapes. Proceed to cook for 2-3 mins until the glue turns darker.

Sprinkle within the Worcestershire sauce and a small of the lager. Mix and proceed including the beer gradually, blending well after each expansion, keeping the warm moo to create beyond any doubt the blend doesn't bubble.

STEP 2

Warm the barbecue to tall. Expel the pot from the warm and mix through the cheese and lime pickle, proceeding to mix until the cheese has softened. (You'll have to be return the dish to a moo warm to totally liquefy the cheese.) Season with a squeeze of pepper and set aside. Organize the cut bread on a heating plate and gently toast both sides beneath the flame broil, 1-2 mins each side. Spread the cheese sauce over the beat and barbecue for an advance 3-4 mins until bubbling and browned. Take off to stand for 2 mins sometime recently serving with a green serving of mixed greens in a lemony dressing, on the off chance that you like.

Fixings

25g unsalted butter

25g plain flour

1 tsp mustard powder

½ tsp Worcestershire sauce

120ml brew

100g develop cheddar, ground

2 tbsp lime pickle, finely chopped

2 thick cuts bread (we utilized sourdough)

green serving of mixed greens, to serve

**Falafel burgers
Strategy**

STEP 1

Deplete the chickpeas and pat dry with kitchen paper. Tip into a nourishment processor in conjunction with the onion, garlic, parsley, cumin, coriander, harissa glue, flour and a small salt. Mix until decently smooth, at that point shape into four patties along with your hands.

STEP 2

Heat the sunflower oil in a non-stick broiling container, and broil the burgers for 3 mins on each side until gently brilliant. Serve with the toasted pitta bread, tomato salsa and green serving of mixed greens.

Fixings

400g can chickpeas, washed and depleted

1 little ruddy onion, generally chopped

1 garlic clove, chopped

modest bunch of flat-leaf parsley or wavy parsley

1 tsp ground cumin

1 tsp ground coriander

½ tsp harissa glue or chilli powder

2 tbsp plain flour

2 tbsp sunflower oil

toasted pitta bread, to serve

200g tub tomato salsa, to serve

green serving of mixed greens, to serve

Smoked salmon, quinoa & dill lunch pot

Strategy

STEP 1

To begin with, make the dressing. Blend the soured cream and lemon juice together in a bowl, at that point include most of the dill, saving a quarter for serving.

STEP 2

In another bowl, combine the quinoa with the cucumber and radishes, and mix through half the dressing. Season and best with the salmon and the rest of the dill.

STEP 3

Put the other half of the dressing in a little pot and sprinkle over the quinoa fair some time recently serving.

Ingredients

2 tbsp half-fat soured cream

2 tbsp lemon juice

½ pack dill, finely chopped

250g pocket ready-to-eat quinoa (we utilized Vendor Gourmet)

½ cucumber, split and cut

4 radishes, finely cut

100g smoked salmon, torn into strips

Prawn & mango serving of mixed greens Strategy

STEP 1

Blend the avocado with the lemon juice, at that point hurl with the prawns, mango, tomatoes, cucumber, spinach and mint. Pack into a lunchbox and sprinkle over the sweet chilli sauce, at that point chill until prepared to eat.

Fixings

½ avocado, peeled and cut into 3d shapes, see tip, underneath cleared out

squeeze of lemon juice

50g little cooked prawns

1 mango cheek, peeled and cut into 3d shapes

4 cherry tomatoes, divided

finger-sized piece cucumber, chopped

modest bunch baby spinach leaves

couple of mint takes off, exceptionally finely destroyed

1-2 tsp sweet chilli sauce

Chorizo & chickpea soup
Strategy

STEP 1

Put a medium skillet on the warm and tip within the tomatoes, taken after by a can of water. Though the tomatoes are warming, quickly cleave the chorizo into thick pieces (removing any skin) and shred the cabbage.

r

STEP 2

Heap the chorizo and cabbage into the skillet with the chilli pieces and chickpeas, at that point disintegrate within the stock 3d shape. Blend well, cover and take off to bubble over a tall warm for 6 mins or until the cabbage is fair delicate. Scoop into bowls and eat with dried up or garlic bread.

Fixings

400g can chopped tomato

110g pack of chorizo wiener (unsliced)

140g wedge Savoy cabbage

sprinkling dried chilli chips

410g can chickpea, depleted and flushed

1 chicken or vegetable stock 3d shape

dried up bread or garlic bread, to serve

Veggie noodle pot

Strategy

STEP 1

To form the omelet, warm the olive oil in a little non-stick broiling container. Include a sprinkle of drain to the beaten eggs, at that point tip into the container. Blend once and permit to cook over a tender warm until nearly set. Flip (employing a plate on the off chance that necessary) and cook on the other side until cooked through. Tip onto a board and cut into strips. (You'll roll the omelet up and cut cuts to allow you spirals, in the event that you like.)

STEP 2

Cook the noodles taking after pack instructions. Deplete and wash beneath cold water, at that point set aside. In the interim, blend the dressing fixings together. Whiten the peas and sugar snap peas, at that point deplete and run beneath cold water to halt them cooking any advance.

STEP 3

To amass the serving of mixed greens, blend the noodles with the infant corn, spring onion, ruddy pepper and green veg, at that point hurl with the dressing and best with strips of omelet.

Fixings

100g noodles (rice, soba or egg)

3 tbsp solidified peas

modest bunch sugar snap peas or mangetout, halved lengthways

modest bunch child corn, divided lengthways

1 spring onion, cut

½ ruddy pepper, deseeded and chopped

For the dressing

1 tbsp reduced-salt soy sauce

1 tsp clear nectar

½ garlic clove, pulverized

juice 1/2 lemon

grinding of new ginger (discretionary)

For the omelette

1 tbsp olive oil

sprinkle of milk

2 eggs, beaten

Storecupboard pasta serving of mixed greens

Method

STEP 1

Blend the onion, capers, pesto and oil. Chip the fish into a bowl with the pasta and tomatoes, at that point blend within the pesto blend.

Ingredients

2 tsp finely chopped ruddy onion

1 tsp caper

1 tbsp pesto

2 tsp olive oil

185g can of fish in spring water, depleted

100g extra pasta shapes

3 sundried tomatoes, chopped

**Classic waffles
Strategy**

STEP 1

Split the egg (for fluffier waffles, utilize as it were the yolk at this arrange) into a large bowl, at that point tip within the flour and a liberal squeeze of salt. Add the sugar, on the off chance that utilizing, at that point slowly whisk within the drain taken after by the liquefied butter until smooth. Whisk within the vanilla, in the event that utilizing. In case you've chosen to form fluffier waffles, whisk the egg white to delicate crests, at that point tenderly overlap this into the player. Then again, make the player by blitzing all the fixings together utilizing a blender or hand blender. Can be made 1-2 hrs. ahead and chilled.

STEP 2

Warm a waffle creator following the manufacturer's enlightening, brush with a small of the oil, at that point scoop in sufficient player to fair cover the surface. Cook taking after the manufacturer's instructions (usually 5-6 mins) until the waffles are brilliant brown and crisp. Serve quickly or keep warm in a moo broiler whereas you make the rest. Sprinkle with maple syrup or sprinkle with icing sugar, on the off chance that you like.

Fixings

1 egg

225g self-rising flour

1 tbsp brilliant caster sugar (discretionary)

250ml drain

50g butter, softened and cooled

½ tsp vanilla extricate (discretionary)

1 tbsp sunflower or vegetable oil

maple syrup and icing sugar, to serve (discretionary)

Chocolate orange waffles
Method

STEP 1

Warm a waffle producer, or if you don't have one, utilize a griddle dish (see tip, underneath). In the meantime, blend the eggs and drain in a container.

STEP 2

Combine the flour, cocoa and sugar in a bowl, at that point slowly whisk in the egg and drain blend until there are no lumps. Gradually pour within the liquefied butter, still whisking, then add the orange substance, pizzazz and chocolate.

STEP 3

Pour a ladleful of the hitter into the waffle press or griddle pan (see underneath), and cook for 5-6 mins, at that point rehash – don't stress in the event that the waffles see dull, it's basically the cocoa. Cut in half and beat with the oranges, maple syrup, more chocolate and whipped cream.

Fixings

2 eggs

200ml drain

130g self-raising flour, sieved

20g cocoa powder, sieved

20g caster sugar

60g butter, liquefied

1 tsp orange substance

1 expansive orange, zested

25g dim chocolate, roughly chopped, also additional to serve

To serve

portioned, maple syrup, ground chocolate and whipped cream

Bubble waffles

Method

STEP 1

Whisk all the waffle ingredients together in an expansive bowl with a pinch of salt until you have got a smooth player. Cover and take off to rest in the ice chest for 1 hr, at that point exchange to a container.

STEP 2

Brush the bubble waffle skillet with a small oil, then set over a medium warm. Once hot, pour in half the player, filling each gap equitably. Join the top of the waffle dish, near and quickly flip over. Cook for 1 1/2-2 mins each side until profound brilliant and fresh on the exterior. Utilize a palette cut to lift the waffle absent from the container and set aside to cool whereas you make the moment one.

STEP 3

Roll the waffles into a cone shape and put in a glass to stand upright. Fill each one with a couple of scoops of ice cream, sprinkle over the sauce and scramble over the raspberries.

Fixings

120g self-rising flour

2 tbsp cornflour

1 tbsp custard powder

100g brilliant caster sugar

2 huge eggs, beaten

1 tbsp vegetable oil, furthermore additional for lubing

1 tsp vanilla extricate

50ml dissipated milk

To serve

matcha green tea ice cream (or any other enhance you like)

dull chocolate sauce

freeze-dried raspberries

Marmite eggs benedict with waffles

Strategy

STEP 1

Warm the waffle producer taking after manufacturer's instructions. Whisk 1 egg white to hardened crests. In a partitioned bowl, combine the flour, bicarb and 1/2 tsp salt. Include the egg yolk, softened butter and drain, and whisk to a smooth, thick hitter. Blend in the cheese, at that point carefully overlap within the egg white.

STEP 2

Warm broiler to 180C/160C fan/gas 4. Utilize a scoop to pour the hitter into the waffle creator and cook for 5 mins. Put the waffles on a heating plate within the broiler for 5 mins to keep warm.

STEP 3

In the meantime, poach the remaining eggs on a moo warm for 3 mins for runny yolks.

STEP 4

Warm the hollandaise sauce taking after pack informational and mix through the Marmite. Top the waffles with two poached eggs, the hollandaise and chives.

Fixings

5 huge eggs, 1 isolated

75g plain flour

squeeze of bicarbonate of pop

½ tbsp butter, softened

150ml entirety drain

50g cheddar, ground

100g hollandaise sauce

2 tsp Marmite

modest bunch chives, cut

**Tomato & pasta soup
Strategy**

STEP 1

Warm 1 tbsp olive oil in an expansive pan. Include the onion and celery and broil for 10-15 mins, or until beginning to mollify, at that point include the garlic and cook for 1 min more. Blend in all the other fixings, but for the pesto and remaining oil, and bring to the bubble.

STEP 2

Decrease the warm and take off to stew for 6-8 mins, or until the pasta is delicate. Season to taste, at that point scoop into bowls.

STEP 3

Blend the remaining oil with the pesto, at that point sprinkle over the soup. Serve with chunks of dried up bread.

Fixings

2 tbsp olive oil

1 onion, chopped

2 celery sticks, chopped

2 garlic cloves, smashed

1 tbsp tomato purée

400g can chopped tomatoes

400g can chickpeas

150g orzo or other little pasta shapes

700ml vegetable stock

2 tbsp basil pesto

dried up bread, to serve

Wiener ragu

Strategy

STEP 1

Warm 2 tbsp of the oil in a pan over a medium warm. Broil the onion with a squeeze of salt for 7 mins. Include the garlic, chilli and rosemary, and cook for 1 min more. Tip within the tomatoes and sugar, and stew for 20 mins.

STEP 2

Warm the remaining oil in a medium searing skillet over a medium warm. Crush the sausagemeat from the skins and sear, breaking it up with a wooden spoon, for 5-7 mins until brilliant. Include to the sauce with the drain and lemon pizzazz, at that point stew for an encourage 5 mins. To solidify, take off to cool totally and exchange to expansive freezerproof sacks.

STEP 3

Cook the pasta taking after pack informational. Deplete and hurl with the sauce. Scramble over the parmesan and parsley takes off to serve.

Fixings

3 tbsp olive oil

1 onion, finely chopped

2 huge garlic cloves, smashed

¼ tsp chilli chips

2 rosemary sprigs, clears out finely chopped

2 x 400g cans chopped tomatoes

1 tbsp brown sugar

6 pork wieners

150ml entirety drain

1 lemon, zested

350g rigatoni pasta

ground parmesan and ½ little bunch parsley, takes off generally chopped, to serve

Fast lentil coconut curry

Strategy

STEP 1

Put the onion, garlic, chilli, carrot and ginger in a nourishment processor and barrage to a smooth glue.

STEP 2

Warm the oil in a medium pan over a medium warm and cook the veg glue for 4-5 mins until fragrant and beginning to mellow. Include the curry glue and cook for 1 min more, at that point include the lentils and mix to combine.

STEP 3

Pour within the coconut drain and 150ml water, and bring to the bubble. Decrease the warm to a stew and cook for 10 mins until thickened and creamy. Add the peas within the last 5 mins, and season well.

STEP 4

Blend in most of the coriander, at that point isolate the curry between four bowls beside the rice. Sprinkle over the remaining coriander and best with the yogurt to serve.

Fixings

1 onion, generally chopped

2 garlic cloves, generally chopped

1 ruddy or green chilli, generally chopped

1 carrot, generally chopped

10g piece of ginger, peeled and chopped

1 tsp vegetable oil

1 ½ tbsp tikka masala curry glue

400g can cooked green lentils

220ml light coconut drain

200g solidified peas

10g coriander, generally chopped

200g cooked brown rice

4 tbsp light coconut or common yogurt, to serve

Spaghetti puttanesca Strategy

STEP 1

Warm the oil in a non-stick skillet over a medium-low warm. Include the onion together with a liberal squeeze of salt and sear for 10 mins, or until delicate. Include the garlic and chilli, on the off chance that utilizing, and cook for a encourage diminutive.

STEP 2

Mix the tomatoes, anchovies, olives and capers into the onion, bring to a tender stew and cook, revealed, for 15 mins. Season to taste.

STEP 3

In the meantime, bring an expansive dish of salted water to the bubble. Cook the spaghetti taking after pack informational, at that point deplete and hurl with the sauce and parsley.

Fixings

3 tbsp olive oil

1 onion, finely chopped

2 huge garlic cloves, smashed

½ tsp chilli drops (discretionary)

400g can chopped tomatoes

5 anchovy filets, finely chopped

120g set dark olives

2 tbsp capers, depleted

300g dried spaghetti

½ little bunch of parsley, finely chopped

Coconut angle curry & rice Strategy

STEP 1

Tip the angle into an expansive bowl with include ½ tsp each of salt and bounty of crisply ground dark pepper, half the lime juice and half the turmeric. Mix delicately to combine. Set aside.

STEP 2

Warm the oil in a singing dish over a medium warm and cook the onion until mellowed, almost 8-10 mins. Include the ginger, garlic, ½ tsp salt, the flavors and remaining turmeric, and cook for 2 mins more until fragrant. Blend within the tomato purée and cook for a miniature more, mixing. Tip the butternut squash and sweet potato blend into a heatproof bowl with a sprinkle of water, cover and microwave on tall for 3 mins until the veg is fork-tender. Tip the blend into the dish with the onion and flavors, and blend to combine.

STEP 3

Include the coconut drain, 180ml water, the tamarind glue, in the event that utilizing, and a squeeze each of salt and dark pepper, and stew over a medium warm for 10-12 mins until thickened and fragrant.

STEP 4

Include the marinated angle to the hot coconut sauce within the dish and cook for 4-6 mins until the angle is misty and cooked through. Break it into chunky drops with a wooden spoon because it cooks. Eliminate the curry from the warm, mix inside the leftover lime squeeze and diffuse with the new coriander, by then serve in a flash with rice.

Fixings

250g solidified economical white angle, cut into bite-sized pieces

1 lime, juiced

1 tsp ground turmeric

3 tbsp vegetable oil or ghee

1 expansive onion, finely chopped

1 tbsp ground ginger

3 garlic cloves, meagerly cut

2 tsp ground cumin

2 tsp ground coriander

½-1 tsp chilli drops or powder, or to taste

2 tbsp tomato purée

250g arranged diced butternut squash and sweet potato blend

200ml coconut drain

2 tbsp tamarind glue (discretionary)

little bunch of coriander, generally chopped, or utilize mint

cooked rice, to serve (roughly 250g crude weight)

Stir-fried meat with ginger

Strategy

STEP 1

Hurl the strips of steak, the lemongrass, soy sauce, half the angle sauce, half the sugar and half the chilli drops together in a bowl. Set aside within the cooler to marinate for at slightest 20 mins or up to 6 hrs.

STEP 2

Blend the remaining angle sauce with the lime juice, remaining chilli pieces, the rest of the sugar and 3 tbsp water, at that point set aside.

STEP 3

Warm 1 tbsp vegetable oil in a huge non-stick or cast press wok or singing dish over a tall warm. Once hot, tip in half the marinated steak strips and stir-fry for 2 mins until fair cooked through, at that point evacuate to a huge plate utilizing tongs or an opened spoon and rehash utilizing another 1 tbsp of oil and the remaining meat. Evacuate to the plate, at that point wipe the wok or skillet clean utilizing kitchen paper.

STEP 4

Include the remaining oil to the skillet and sear the green pepper and the white parts of the spring onion. Stir-fry over a tall warm for 2-3 mins, at that point include the garlic and ginger and stir-fry for another 45 seconds-1 min. Return the steak to the skillet, mix well, at that point include the lime dressing and most of the basil clears out, blending well to coat.

STEP 5

Separate the stir-fry between bowls nearby rice or noodles, at that point diffuse with the chopped peanuts, the remaining basil leaves and the green parts of the spring onions.

Fixings

350g incline hamburger, cut over the grain into lean cuts (you would like a quick-cooking cut, such as diminutive steak)

1 lemongrass stalk, trimmed and finely chopped

1 tbsp soy sauce

2 tbsp angle sauce

4 tsp brown sugar

½ tsp chilli pieces

1 lime, juiced

3 tbsp vegetable oil

1 green pepper, meagerly cut

2 bunches of spring onions, green and white parts isolated and finely cut

6 garlic cloves, finely chopped

1 tbsp ground ginger

little bunch of basil, or purple basil, takes off picked and generally chopped

cooked rice (almost 250g raw weight), or cooked rice noodles

50g broiled peanuts, generally chopped

**Lemon & greens pesto pasta
Strategy**

STEP 1

Cook the pasta taking after pack enlightening. In the meantime, cook the broccoli for 4 mins in bubbling salted water. Deplete, at that point put in a food processor in conjunction with the basil, spinach and pine nuts. Pulse until combined.

STEP 2

Blend within the garlic, lemon get-up-and-go and juice, olive oil, peas, parmesan and delicate cheese, and season to taste.

STEP 3

Deplete the pasta, saving a small of the cooking water. Return the pasta to the skillet and include the pesto beside a sprinkle of water to extricate. Hurl together, check the flavoring and serve.

Fixings

350g pasta (we utilized linguine)

½ little head of broccoli, cut into florets

expansive modest bunch of basil

1 huge modest bunch of spinach shriveled in bubbling water, cooled and abundance water crushed out

4 tbsp pine nuts

1 garlic clove, ground

½ lemon, zested and juiced

6 tbsp additional virgin olive oil

expansive modest bunch of solidified peas, set aside in bubbled water until warmed through

3 tbsp ground parmesan or veggie lover difficult cheese

3 tbsp delicate cheese

Shelled nut butter chicken

Strategy

STEP 1

Warm 1 tbsp of the oil in a profound singing dish over a medium heat. Brown the chicken in clusters, setting aside once brilliant. Broil the onion for 8 minutes until relaxed. At that point include the garlic, chilli and ginger and fry within the other 1 tbsp oil for 1 min. Include the garam masala and sear for 1 min more.

STEP 2

Mix in the shelled nut butter, coconut drain and tomatoes, and bring to a stew. Return the chicken to the dish and include the chopped coriander. Cook for 30 minutes, or until the chicken is cooked through and the sauce has thickened.

STEP 3

Serve with the remaining coriander, simmered peanuts and rice, in the event that you like.

Fixings

2tbsp avocado oil

8 skinless boneless chicken thighs, cut into chunks

1 onion, finely chopped

3 garlic cloves, smashed

2 ruddy chillies, finely cut (deseeded in case you do not like it as well hot)

2tsp new ginger, ground

2tbsp garam masala

100g smooth shelled nut butter

400ml coconut drain

400g can chopped tomatoes

coriander, ½ generally chopped, ½ takes off picked

simmered peanuts, to serve

cauliflower rice to serve

**Pork & apple burgers
Method**

STEP 1

Separate the sausagemeat into four parcels and shape into patties. Sear in a non-stick dish for 10-12 mins, flipping a couple of times, until brilliant on both sides and cooked all the way through.

STEP 2

Warm barbecue to high. Slice the buns in half and toast beneath the flame broil, cut-side up.

STEP 3

Spread the foot parts of the toasted buns with the preserves, at that point include the burgers, apple cuts, rocket, mayonnaise and mustard (if utilizing). Beat with the bun tops and serve nearby sweet potato wedges, on the off chance that you like.

Fixings

300g sausagemeat

4 whole meal burger buns

4 tsp onion jelly

2 apples, cored and daintily cut

2 modest bunches rocket

2 tsp mayonnaise

a small English mustard (discretionary)

sweet potato wedges, to serve (discretionary)

Messy joes

Strategy

STEP 1

Warm the oil in a profound searing skillet, and tip within the mince, breaking it up with a wooden spoon as you go, until browned all over. Mix within the onion and pepper and cook for 8-10 mins until mollified. Tip within the tomatoes and Nando's PERi-BBQ sauce, and season. Stew for 20-25 mins until the sauce has thickened.

STEP 2

Put the cheese cuts on best of the mince and cover with a top for 2 mins to let it soften into the sauce. Heap into the buns with the firm onions, and lettuce on the side for scooping up the additional sauce.

Fixings

1tbsp vegetable oil

1 onion, finely chopped

2 little ruddy peppers or yellow peppers, finely chopped

400g minced hamburger

2 x 400g cans chopped tomatoes

4tbsp Nando's PERi-BBQ sauce

4 cheese cuts

6 burger buns

fresh onions, to serve

tbsp ice sheet lettuce, to serve

low-cooker pumpkin soup

Strategy

STEP 1

Warm the oil in a huge dish over a medium warm and sear the onions and ginger for 10 mins, mixing every so often until relaxed and beginning to colour. Mix within the garlic, curry powder, ground coriander and dried chillies, on the off chance that utilizing, and cook for 1 min more.

STEP 2

Tip the blend into a large moderate cooker together with all the remaining fixings, but the new coriander. Include 2 liters' water. Cook for 8 hrs. on tall, or overnight for 15 hrs. on moo. Mix well, at that point barrage employing a hand blender until smooth. Scoop into bowls and diffuse over the new coriander to serve. Once totally cool, the soup will keep chilled in a sealed shut holder for 48 hrs. or solidified for up to two months. Warm in a container over a moo warm or within the microwave until channeling hot.

Fixings

2 tbsp rapeseed oil

3 onions (480g), chopped

30g ginger, peeled and chopped

3 huge garlic cloves, chopped

1½-2 tbsp medium curry powder

1 tsp ground coriander

½ tsp pulverized dried chillies (discretionary)

1kg pumpkin or butternut squash (substance as it were), cut into 3d shapes

1 tbsp vegetable bouillon powder (guarantee veggie lover, in the event that required)

400g can coconut drain

180g dried ruddy lentils

15g coriander, chopped

Halloumi & watermelon bulgur serving of mixed greens

Strategy

STEP 1

Bubble the pot. Put the bulgur wheat in a bowl with a few flavoring, pour over sufficient hot water to fair cover, at that point cover with cling film and set aside to assimilate the fluid whereas you get ready the remaining fixings.

STEP 2

Heat an expansive searing skillet and include the pumpkin seeds, toast for a couple of mins until the seeds begin to crackle and pop, at that point tip into a dish and set aside. Warm a sprinkle of oil within the skillet. Include the halloumi cuts and sear for 2-3 mins on each side or until brilliant.

STEP 3

Unwrap the bulgur wheat and check that it is delicate (on the off chance that not, re-cover and take off for another 5 mins). All the water ought to have been ingested, but on the off chance that not, deplete the abundance. Incorporate the excess oil, the cucumber, spices, lemon outfit and-go and squeeze, and pumpkin seeds to the bulgur wheat and throw well. Exchange to a platter, beat with the watermelon and halloumi, and diffuse with the saved herbs.

Fixings

200g bulgur wheat

50g pumpkin seed

3 tbsp olive or rapeseed oil

250g pack halloumi cheese, cut into 10-12 cuts

1 cucumber, split lengthways, seeds scooped out and cut into chunks

expansive bunch either parsley, mint, coriander or basil, or a blend, chopped, saving a couple of takes off to serve

get-up-and-go and juice 2 lemons

14 watermelons, chopped up, or a 400g ready-made pack

**Kedgeree with poached egg
Strategy**

STEP 1

Cook the rice taking after pack instructions, then deplete and set aside. In the meantime, warm 1 tbsp of the oil in a non-stick searing container and cook the onion and garlic for 5 mins. Hurl the angle pieces with the curry powder and remaining oil. Include to the dish. Cook for another 5 mins, mixing carefully and turning the angle.

STEP 2

Include the rice to the container and turn up the warm, at that point mix well (the angle will break up a small). Cook for 1-2 mins, at that point mix within the lemon and parsley. Turn the heat down as moo because it will go, and put on a cover.

STEP 3

Bring a container of water to the bubble, turn down the warm and poach the eggs. Season the kedgeree and split between plates, finishing off each with a poached egg.

Fixings

300g long grain rice

2 tbsp olive oil

1 onion, finely chopped

2 garlic cloves, finely chopped

390g pack angle pie mix, defrosted in case solidified

1 piled tbsp gentle or medium curry powder

juice 1 lemon

¼ little pack parsley, chopped

4 eggs

Chicken alfredo

Strategy

STEP 1

Warm the olive oil in a non-stick broiling skillet over a medium tall warm. Include the chicken thighs and sear for around 10 mins, turning half way, until they are brilliant brown and cooked through. Set aside to cool a small, at that point utilize two forks to shred.

STEP 2

Bring a container of salted water to the bubble and include the pasta, cook for 1 diminutive less that bundle enlightening. While the pasta is cooking, include the butter to the singing dish over a medium warm, scratching the bottom a small to urge any of the browned bits. Tip within the cream alongside the nutmeg and bring to a stew. Include the chicken back to the pan.

STEP 3

Once the pasta is cooked, utilize tongs to transfer the pasta straight from the water into the frying pan with the cream blend. Sprinkle most of the parmesan over and utilize the tongs to hurl it all together, including a sprinkle of the pasta water on the off chance that it looks a small hardened. Season well, at that point tip into bowls. Best with the remaining parmesan, a diffusing of parsley, and dark pepper.

Fixings

1 tbsp olive oil

4 skinless boneless chicken thighs, cut down the middle

300g fettuccine, or tagliatelle

1 tbsp butter

200ml twofold cream

½ a nutmeg, ground

100g parmesan

parsley, chopped, to serve

Big-batch bolognese

Strategy

STEP 1

Warm the oil in a really huge pan. Tenderly cook the bacon, onions, carrots and celery for

20 mins until brilliant. Include the garlic, herbs, narrows and mushrooms, at that point cook for 2 mins more.

STEP 2

Warm an expansive singing dish until really hot. Crumble in fair sufficient mince to cover the dish, cook until brown, at that point tip in with the veg. Continue to broil the mince in clusters until utilized up. Tip the tomatoes and purée in with the mince and veg. Wash the cans out with the red wine, on the off chance that you have got some, or with a small water, at that point include to the dish with the vinegar and sugar. Season liberally and bring to a stew. Stew slowly for 1 hr until thick and insolent and the mince is delicate. Serve with pasta and parmesan.

STEP 3

On the off chance that you want to make this in a moderate cooker, visit our moderate cooker bolognese formula.

Fixings

4 tbsp olive oil

6 smoked bacon rashers, chopped

4 onions, finely chopped

3 carrots, finely chopped

4 celery sticks, finely chopped

8 garlic cloves, smashed

2 tbsp dried blended herbs

2 cove clears out

500g mushrooms, sliced

1½ kg incline minced hamburger (or utilize half meat, half pork mince)

6 x 400g cans chopped tomatoes

6 tbsp tomato purée

expansive glass ruddy wine (discretionary)

4 tbsp ruddy wine vinegar

1 tbsp sugar

parmesan, to serve

Five-bean chilli

Method

STEP 1

Warm the oil in a casserole dish and broil the onion and peppers for 10 mins over a medium warm until the onion is brilliant brown. Add the garlic and flavors, and broil for 1 min. Pour within the tomatoes, both cans of beans, 50ml water, at that point include the sugar and season. Stew, blending frequently, for 15-20 mins until thickened.

STEP 2

In the meantime, cook the rice taking after pack instructions. Serve the chilli on the rice and scramble over the coriander. Best with a spoonful of soured cream, or guacamole, in the event that you like.

Fixings

1½ tbsp rapeseed oil

1 onion, cut

2 peppers, cut

2 garlic cloves, pulverized

1 tbsp ground cumin

1 tbsp ground coriander

2 tsp hot smoked paprika

400g can chopped tomatoes

400g can blended beans, depleted

400g can dark beans, depleted

squeeze of sugar

250g brown rice

½ small bunch coriander, chopped

soured cream or guacamole, to serve (optional)

Small fiery veggie pies Strategy

STEP 1

To create the topping, bubble the potatoes for 15-20 mins until delicate then drain, reserving the water, and squash with the ground and fresh coriander and yogurt until creamy.

STEP 2

Whereas the potatoes are boiling, heat the oil in a huge dish, include the ginger and sear briefly, tip within the curry powder and garlic, mixing rapidly as you do not need it to burn, at that point tip in a can of chickpeas with the water from the can. Mix well, at that point pound within the container to crush them up a bit, at that point tip within the moment can of chickpeas, again with the water from the can, together with the carrots, corn, bouillon and tomato purée. Stew for 5-10 mins, including a few of the potato water, in case required, to release.

STEP 3

Warm the stove to 200C/180C fan/gas 6. Spoon the filling into four-person pie dishes (each around 10cm wide, 8cm profound) and best with the pound, smoothing it to seal circular the edges of the dishes. On the off chance that you're taking after our Solid Eat Less Arrange, prepare two for 25 mins until brilliant, and cook half the spinach, sparing the rest of the pack for another day. Cover and chill the leftover two pies to eat one more day Will keep within the cooler for four days – in the event that taking after the Sound Slim down Arrange pop the extra two pies within the cooler for the conclusion of the week. In the event that solidifying, to warm, prepare from solidified for 40-45 mins until brilliant and channeling hot.

Fixings

2 tbsp rapeseed oil

2 tbsp finely chopped ginger

3 tbsp curry powder

3 garlic cloves, ground

2 x 400g cans chickpeas, undrained

320g carrots, coarsely ground

160g solidified sweetcorn

1 tbsp vegetable bouillon powder

4 tbsp tomato purée

250g spinach, cooked

For the topping

750g potatoes, peeled and cut into 3cm chunks

1 tsp ground coriander

10g new coriander, chopped

150g coconut yogurt

Essential lentils

Strategy

STEP 1

Liquefy 1 tbsp coconut oil in an expansive pan. Include the onion and a squeeze of salt, and cook for 8 mins. Blend within the garlic and ginger and cook for a couple of mins more. Include the lentils, turmeric and tomatoes, mix to combine, at that point pour in 1 litre of water. Bring to the bubble, at that point turn down and stew for 25-30 mins, blending sometimes, until the lentils are delicate.

STEP 2

Warm the rest of the oil in a broiling dish. When it's exceptionally hot, include the flavors and broil for a min or so until fragrant, at that point mix them through. Include the lemon juice and season to taste. Will keep for four days within the ice chest, or solidify it in bunches and utilize to create our lentil kedgeree, lentil squanders, or spinach dhal with harissa yogurt.

Fixings

2 tbsp coconut oil

2 onions, chopped

4 garlic cloves, chopped

expansive piece of ginger, chopped

300g ruddy part lentils

1 tsp turmeric

2 tomatoes, generally chopped

1 tsp coriander seeds

1 tsp cumin seeds

1 tsp dark mustard seeds

1 lemon, juiced

Urad dhal

Strategy

STEP 1

Wash the dhal in at least three changes of cold water until the water runs clear. Put the flushed dhal in a huge bowl with bounty of cold water, cover and take off to douse at room temperature for 12-24 hrs.

STEP 2

Deplete and wash the dhal, at that point tip into a huge pan. Cover with 2 litres of cold water and bring to the bubble, skimming any froth from the beat. Turn down the warm, half-cover and tenderly stew for 2½-3 hrs. In case the water level begins to drop underneath the best of the dhal, include a splash more bubbling water. Once cooked, the dhal ought to be completely soft and begin breaking down into the fluid. In the event that the fluid is still lean, stew for an additional few mins and squash the dhal delicately to assist thicken.

STEP 3

Warm the oil in a little singing container. Include the garlic and ginger and broil delicately for 1-2 mins to mollify but not brown.

Include the ground coriander, chilli powder, turmeric and tomato purée with an expansive sprinkle of water. Cook for 1-2 mins, at that point rub into the dish of dhal and tenderly warm through.

STEP 4

Include additional water if needed to make the dhal looser and rich. Sprinkle over the garam masala and clear from the warm. Serve in bowls with rice topped with a whirl of coconut yogurt, a scrambling of coriander and a few lime wedges on the side for crushing over.

Fixings

250g urad dal (too known as urid beans, dark gram or vegan mungo)

1 tbsp rapeseed oil

5 garlic cloves, smashed

1 tbsp finely ground ginger

1 tbsp ground coriander

2 tsp gentle chilli powder

1 tsp turmeric

2 tbsp tomato purée

1 tsp garam masala

To serve

cooked brown basmati rice

coconut yogurt

little bunch coriander, generally chopped

lime wedges

Italian vegetable soup
Strategy

STEP 1

Tenderly cook the onion, carrots and celery within the oil in a huge pot for 20 mins, until delicate. Sprinkle in water in the event that they adhere. Include the sugar, garlic, purée, herbs and courgettes and cook for 4-5 mins on a medium warm until they brown a small.

STEP 2

Pour within the beans, tomatoes and stock, at that point stew for 20 mins. On the off chance that you're solidifying it, cool and do so presently (solidify for up to three months). On the off chance that not, include half the Parmesan and the pasta and stew for 6-8 mins until pasta cooked. Sprinkle with basil and remaining Parmesan to serve. In case solidified, defrost at that point re-heat some time recently including pasta and cheese and proceeding as over.

Fixings

2 each of onions and carrots, chopped

4 sticks celery, chopped

1 tbsp olive oil

2 tbsp sugar

4 garlic cloves, pulverized

2 tbsp tomato purée

2 narrows take off

few sprigs thyme

3 courgettes, chopped

400g can butter beans, depleted

400g can chopped tomatoes

1.2l vegetable stock

100g parmesan or veggie lover proportionate, ground

140g little pasta shapes

little bunch basil, destroyed

Spiced parsnip & cauliflower soup

Strategy

STEP 1

Warm the oil in an expansive pot and include the vegetables. Cover in part and sweat gradually for 10-15 mins until delicate but not brown. In an isolated skillet, dry-roast the flavors with a squeeze of salt for many mins until fragrant. Pound with a pestle and mortar to a fine powder.

STEP 2

Include the garlic, chilli, ginger and flavors to the vegetables, and cook for approximately 5 mins, blending frequently. Add the lemon get-up-and-go and juice. Pour within the stock, topping up in the event that essential to fair cover the veg. Stew for 25-30 mins until all the vegetables are delicate.

STEP 3

Purée with a blender until smooth. Weaken the consistency with more water in case required, until you get a thick but effortlessly pourable soup. Season liberally, blend within the coriander and include more lemon juice to adjust the taste.

Destroy straight or chill inside the refrigerator to warm. This too solidifies delightfully. Serve with dried up bread, in case you like.

Fixings

1 tbsp olive oil

1 medium cauliflower, cut into florets

3 parsnips, chopped

2 onions, chopped

1 tbsp fennel seed

1 tsp coriander seed

½ tsp turmeric

3 garlic cloves, cut

1-2 green chillies, deseeded and chopped

5cm piece ginger, sliced

get-up-and-go and juice 1 lemon

1l vegetable stock

modest bunch coriander, chopped

Bearings

For the London broil:

Set an expansive resealable plastic sack in a medium pot and drag the edges of the pack over the sides of the skillet for simple get to to the sack. Include the olive oil, Worcestershire sauce, garlic cloves, lemon juice, 1 teaspoon salt and 1 teaspoon pepper to the pack and whisk to combine. Include the London broil and seal the sack firmly. Evacuate the pack from the container and utilize your hands to pivot the meat, coating altogether in the marinade. Lay the pack level on a cutting board and marinate at room temperature for 1 hour, flipping the pack after 30 minutes. (The prepared meat can too be put away within the fridge overnight. Let rest at room temperature for 20 minutes prior to cooking.)

For the gribiche:

In the interim, bring a medium pan filled with water to a bubble over tall warm. Utilize an expansive spoon to delicately include the eggs. Bubble for 10 minutes. Deplete the eggs and wash beneath cold water to halt the cooking. Crack, peel and generally chop the eggs.

Whisk the oil, mustard, vinegar, garlic and 1/2 teaspoon every one of salt and pepper in a medium bowl. Mix within the parsley, chives, capers and cornichons. Overlap within the chopped eggs. Cover and set aside to marinate. (The gribiche can be refrigerated for up to 2 days; return to room temperature some time recently utilizing.)

While the gribiche is marinating, preheat the broiler to high by placing a stove rack 4 inches from the warming element. Cover a rimmed heating sheet with aluminum thwart and put within the broiler to preheat.

Expel the steak from the sack and dispose of any stuck-on garlic cloves. Drag the preheated sheet container from the oven and put the steak in the center. Broil until pleasantly charred and an instant-read thermometer inserted sideways into the center of the steak registers between 120 and 125 degrees F, 6 to 10 minutes depending on thickness. Exchange the steak to the cutting board and let rest for 10 minutes.

For the asparagus:

Whereas the steak rests, include the asparagus to the same sheet skillet and hurl with the olive oil. Season with 1/2 teaspoon salt and 1/4 teaspoon pepper. Broil until the asparagus is energetically green and crisp-tender, around 3 minutes.

Divide the asparagus among the plates and spoon the best with the gribiche.

Fixings

Deselect All

London broil:

2 tablespoons extra-virgin olive oil

2 tablespoons Worcestershire sauce

4 cloves garlic, crushed

Juice of 1 lemon

Legitimate salt and crisply ground black pepper

2 pounds beat circular London broil steak (1/2 inch to 1 inch thick)

Gribiche:

3 huge eggs

1/4 container extra-virgin olive oil

1 tablespoon Dijon mustard

1 tablespoon white wine vinegar

1 clove garlic, ground

Legitimate salt and naturally ground dark pepper

1 container new parsley, finely chopped

2 tablespoons dried chives

1 tablespoon depleted capers, generally chopped

6 cornichons, generally chopped

Asparagus:

2 pounds' pencil-thin asparagus, woody stems evacuated

1 tablespoon extra-virgin olive oil

Kosher salt and crisply ground dark pepper

Parker House Rolls

With a beat layer of broken up spread and a sprinkling of sea salt, these splendid earthy colored Parker House rolls aren't anything brief of prize commendable. Made for the Parker House Hotel in Boston in a little while after it opened in 1855, these exemplary yeast rolls are occasionally called wallet rolls since of their shape, which resembles a handbag:

Fair as perfect for sandwiching a cut of Thanksgiving turkey or occasion ham as they are slathered with nectar or a smooth of stick for breakfast.

In case you're unused to heating bread, supper rolls are a great put to begin, but make beyond any doubt to arrange ahead so there's time to let the mixture rise some time recently you shape it and for the formed buns to chill some time recently heating.

We favor to work this mixture by hand, but feel free to whip them up in a stand blender with a mixture snare in case you'd or maybe. And while some bread formulas prescribe letting the mixture rise in a warm put, this Parker House rolls formula calls for rising at room temperature. Cooler temps will energize the batter to rise more slowly, giving it time to develop flavor. You'll even chill the mixture overnight, at that point shape the rolls the following day.

Fixings

envelope dynamic dry yeast

1

glass entirety drain

¼

container vegetable shortening

3

tablespoons sugar

1½

teaspoons legitimate salt

1

huge egg, room temperature

3½

glasses all-purpose flour, plus more for surface

Canola oil (for bowl)

¼

glass unsalted butter

Step 1

Whisk yeast and ¼ container warm water (110°-115°) in a small bowl; let stand 5 minutes until frothy.

Step 2

Warm milk in a little pan over medium until fair warm. Combine shortening, sugar, and legitimate salt in a huge bowl. Include warm drain; whisk to mix, breaking up shortening into little clumps (it may not liquefy totally). Whisk in yeast blend and egg. Include 3½ glasses flour; stir vigorously with a wooden spoon until batter shapes. Manipulate mixture with gently floured hands on a softly floured work surface until smooth, 4–5 minutes. Transfer to a softly oiled bowl; turn to coat. Cover freely with plastic wrap. Let stand at room temperature until multiplied, approximately 1½ hours.

Step 3

Preheat stove to 350°. Soften butter in a little pot. Delicately brush 13x9" heating dish with a few dissolved butter. Punch down batter; separate into 4 rise to pieces. Working with 1 piece at a time, roll out on a softly floured surface into a 12x6" rectangle.

Step 4

Cut longwise into three 2"-wide strips; cut each crosswise into three 4x2" rectangles. Brush half of each (approximately 2x2") with dissolved butter; fold unbuttered side over, permitting a ¼-inch overhang. Put level in 1 corner of dish, folded edge against brief side of dish. Include remaining rolls, shingling to create 1 long push. Rehash with remaining mixture for 4 lines. Brush with softened butter, freely cover with plastic, and chill at slightest 30 minutes or up to 6 hours.

Step 5

Heat rolls until brilliant and puffed, 25–35 minutes. Brush with butter; sprinkle ocean salt over. Serve warm.

For-the-freezer ratatouille

Strategy

STEP 1

Warm stove to 200C/180C fan/gas 6. Scramble the onions in a broiling tin, season and broil for 25 mins, mixing once in a while, until charred and relaxed. Rehash with the peppers for 20 mins, at that point the courgette for fair 15 mins.

STEP 2

Warm a non-stick searing dish. Cut the aubergines into 2-3cm thick rounds and orchestrate within the pan (only cut what you'll fit in your dish at a time – cooking naturally cut cuts in bunches ought to anticipate them going brown). Cook over a tall warm until charred on both sides, at that point evacuate to a microwave-proof plate. Rehash in clumps until all are pleasantly crisped and browned. Cover the plate with cling film, jab in a few of gaps, at that point microwave the aubergines on Tall for approximately 5 mins until delicate. You'll got to do this in bunches. Quarter the cuts, or cut into chunks. (Because you're singing without oil, they'll burn some time recently they're cooked through, so wrapping up in a microwave is perfect. In case you do not have one, fair include to the sauce for the ultimate 10-15 mins stewing, but they may break up a bit.)

STEP 3

Whereas broiling the veg, put the garlic within the non-stick broiling skillet or a huge skillet with a little glass of water. Stew until the water is nearly gone, at that point tip within the cherry and chopped tomatoes, sugar, vinegar and bounty of flavoring. Stew for 20 mins until thickened and impudent. Taste for flavoring, at that point turn off and combine with the veg. Cool, partition into 10 parcels and solidify.

STEP 4

To serve as Greek veg prepare with feta (serves 1, prep 10 mins, cook 15 mins):

Mix herbs through 1 serving defrosted ratatouille and tip into a little dish. Sprinkle with breadcrumbs, at that point include feta with a pinch more herbs. Heat at 200C/180C fan/gas 6 for 15 mins in case defrosted, or 25-30 mins from frozen. Toss Baby Diamond takes off with spring onion, cucumber and lemon juice. Serve with the heat. Per serving:

236 kcals, protein 13g, carbs 34g, fat 5g, sat fat 3g, fiber 10g, sugar 20g, salt 1.0g

STEP 5

To serve as veggie chilli coats (serves 1, prep 5 mins, cook almost 1hr):

Prepare potato within the oven. Include a number of tbsp water to a dish with cumin seeds and chilli powder. Stew, and fair some time recently the water vanishes, mix in 1 serving of defrosted ratatouille. Warm through, at that point mix in coriander. Split the potato, beat with veggie chilli and Greek yogurt. Serve with rocket clears out dressed with lemon juice. Per serving:

270kcals, protein 14g, carbs 50g, fat 3g, sat fat 0g, fibrew 12g, sugar 20g, salt 0.4g

STEP 6

To serve as tacky stuffed peppers (serves 2, prep 15 mins, cook 20 mins):

Divide peppers down the stalks and rub out any seeds. Separate 1 serving of defrosted ratatouille between the pepper parts. Grind over cheddar, at that point prepare for 15-20 mins at 200C/180C fan/gas 6. Serve with broccoli and spinach tossed with balsamic vinegar. Per serving:

173 kcals, protein 12g, carbs 21g, fat 4g, sat fat 2g, fiber 10g, sugar 20g, salt 0.4g

Fixings

250g ruddy onion, cut into 3cm chunks

250g white onion, cut into 3cm chunks

600g ruddy and yellow pepper - after deseeding and expelling stalks, cut into chunks

1kg courgette, cut into 3cm chunks

1kg aubergine

20g garlic clove, smashed

800g cherry tomato

3 x 400g cans chopped tomatoes

1 tbsp sugar

2 tbsp ruddy wine vinegar

To serve as Greek veg prepare with feta (serves 1)

1 tsp dried thyme or oregano, additionally a squeeze additional

1 tbsp whole meal breadcrumb

25g light feta cheese

30g Small Jewel lettuce takes off

25g cut spring onion

50g cut cucumber

press of lemon juice

To serve as veggie chilli coats (serves 1)

1 little preparing potato weighing 100g

1 tsp cumin seed

1 tsp mellow chilli powder

2 tbsp chopped coriander

25g fat-free Greek yogurt

10g rocket clears out

squeeze of lemon juice

To serve as corny stuffed peppers (serves 2)

2 small peppers of any colour

25g lighter develop cheddar

200g cooked broccoli

20g child spinach clears out

1 tsp balsamic vinegar

Tofu & spinach cannelloni Strategy

STEP 1

Warm half the oil in a pan, add onion and 1/3 of the garlic and sear for 4 mins until softened. Pour in tomatoes, season and bring to the bubble. Reduce heat and cook for 10 mins until sauce thickens.

STEP 2

Warm half remaining oil in a broiling dish and cook another 1/3 of garlic for 1 min, at that point include half the pine nuts and the spinach. Shrivel spinach, at that point tip out abundance fluid. Evacuate from the warm; permit to cool somewhat.

STEP 3

Warm stove to 200C/180C fan/gas 6. Empty half pureed tomatoes into a 20 x 30cm dish. Partition spinach blend between lasagne sheets, roll up and lay on beat of sauce. Pour over remaining sauce. Prepare for 30 mins.

STEP 4

Blend crumbs with remaining garlic and pine nuts. Sprinkle over best of dish, sprinkle with remaining oil and heat for 10 mins until scraps are brilliant.

Fixings

2 tbsp olive oil

1 onion, chopped

3 garlic cloves, finely chopped

2 x 400g cans chopped tomatoes

50g pine nuts, generally chopped

400g sack spinach

squeeze ground nutmeg

349g pack smooth tofu

300g pack new lasagne sheets

4 tbsp new breadcrumbs

Sheep stew with feathery rosemary & cheddar dumplings

Strategy

STEP 1

Season the sheep pieces and hurl within the flour. Warm 1 tbsp of the oil in a huge flameproof casserole dish over a medium-high warm and brown half the sheep pieces, guaranteeing they're profoundly coloured some time recently turning over to brown on all sides. Expel to a bowl. Rehash with the remaining oil and the rest of the sheep pieces. Use caution not to pack the skillet, or the sheep will steam instead of brown.

STEP 2

Sear the bacon within the container for many minutes, at that point tip within the veg and garlic. Cook for 3-4 mins more until the veg has fair begun to mollify, at that point blend within the browned sheep, the pearl grain, rosemary, tomato purée, Worcestershire sauce, redcurrant jam and stock. Season well, at that point tuck the narrows clears out into the sauce. Bring to a stew.

STEP 3

Cut out a circle of preparing parchment that's large sufficient to cover the stew (typically called a cartouche, and it makes a difference keep the meat submerged within the stew). Put this straightforwardly on the surface of the stew, at that point cover with the top and turn the warm to moo. Stew for 1 hr 30 mins-2 hrs., or until the meat is delicate but not falling separated. On the other hand, exchange to a moderate cooker for 6-8 hrs. on moo. Once cooled, will keep solidified for up to six months.

STEP 4

In the interim, make the dumplings. Weigh the flour out into a bowl and include the heating powder and ½ tsp salt. Stir within the rosemary and half the cheddar. Make a well within the middle and tip in the yogurt, at that point blend to firm but malleable batter, including a sprinkle of water in the event that it feels as well dry. Separate the mixture into 12 break even with pieces and roll into balls. Chill until required.

STEP 5

Warm the stove to 180C/160C fan/gas 4. Evacuate the stew from the warm, dispose of the cartouche and organize the dumplings on best of the stew. Cover with the top, exchange to the broiler and cook for 20 mins. Remove the cover and sprinkle the rest of the cheddar over the dumplings. Cook for 10-15 mins more, revealed, until the dumplings have browned and puffed up.

Fixings

600g boneless bear or leg of sheep, goat, lamb or hogget, trimmed of abundance fat and cut into 3cm pieces

2 tbsp plain flour

2 tbsp neutral-tasting oil

75g smoked bacon lardons or pancetta

2 onions, chopped

2 carrots, cut into 2cm chunks

2 celery sticks, cut

2 garlic cloves, pulverized

75g pearl grain

2 rosemary branches, needles picked and finely hacked

1 tbsp tomato purée

1 tbsp Worcestershire sauce

1 tbsp redcurrant jam

650ml chicken or lamb stock

2 cove leaves

For the dumplings

175g self-rising flour

1 tsp baking powder

2 rosemary branches, needles picked and finely hacked

50g cheddar, grated

100g full-fat common yogurt

Overnight oats

Strategy

STEP 1

The night some time recently serving, mix the cinnamon and 100ml water (or drain) into your oats with a squeeze of salt.

STEP 2

The another day, extricate with a small more water (or drain) in case required. Best with the yogurt, berries, a sprinkle of nectar and the nut butter.

Fixings

¼ tsp ground cinnamon

50g rolled porridge oats

2 tbsp common yogurt

50g blended berries

sprinkle of nectar

½ tbsp nut butter (we utilized almond)

Prepared oats

Strategy

STEP 1

In case you're cooking them within the broiler, warm it to 180C/160C fan/gas 4. Put the oats in a blender and beat multiple times until they start to take after flour. Include the heating powder, chopped banana, maple syrup or nectar, eggs and blended flavor or cinnamon, and whizz until smooth. Mix within the chocolate chips or berries.

STEP 2

In case utilizing an air-fryer instead of a broiler, warm the discuss fryer to 180C for 4 mins. Delicately oil four heatproof ramekins, at that point partition the player between them. Heat for 8-10 mins within the air-fryer or 20-25 mins within the stove until well-risen and the prepared oats spring back when gently squeezed. Diffuse with more chocolate chips or berries some time recently serving, in case you like.

Fixings

100g porridge oats

1 tsp preparing powder

1 banana, peeled and chopped

1 tbsp maple syrup or nectar

2 eggs

squeeze of blended flavor or ground cinnamon

100g chocolate chips, blueberries or raspberries, also additional to serve

flavorless oil, for the ramekins

American hotcakes
Method

STEP 1

Blend 200g self-rising flour, 1 ½ tsp preparing powder, 1 tbsp golden caster sugar and a squeeze of salt together in a huge bowl.

STEP 2

Make a well within the middle with the back of your spoon at that point include 3 expansive eggs, 25g dissolved butter and 200ml drain.

STEP 3

Whisk together either with a swell whisk or electric hand mixers until smooth at that point pour into a container.

STEP 4

Warm a little handle of butter and 1 tsp of oil in a large, non-stick singing skillet over a medium warm. When the butter looks foamy, pour in rounds of the hitter, around 8cm wide. Make beyond any doubt you do not put the flapjacks as well near together as they will spread amid cooking. Cook the hotcakes on one side for approximately 1-2 mins or until parcels of little bubbles begin to seem and pop on the surface. Flip the flapjacks over and cook for a encourage diminutive on the other side. Rehash until all the hitter is utilized up.

STEP 5

Serve your flapjacks stacked up on a plate with a sprinkle of maple syrup and any of your top choice garnishes.

Fixings

200g self-rising flour

1 ½ tsp preparing powder

1 tbsp golden caster sugar

3 huge eggs

25g liquefied butter, additionally additional for cooking

200ml drain

vegetable oil, for cooking

To serve

maple syrup

fixings of your choice, such as cooked bacon, chocolate chips, blueberries or shelled nut butter and stick

Turbo beans & cheese on toast

Strategy

STEP 1

Warm the oil in a heavy-based frying skillet over a medium heat and sear the onion for 8-10 mins until relaxed and marginally caramelised. Include the garlic and flavors, the chipotle chilli glue or chilli pieces, in case utilizing, and a few flavoring. Broil for a number of minutes more until the blend is fragrant.

STEP 2

Include the tomatoes, at that point whirl out the container utilizing 100ml water and include this as well. Stew for 10-15 mins until the mixture has thickened. Rush the sauce employing a hand blender, at that point taste for flavoring. Tip within the beans and blend well to coat. Warm through over a medium warm for 5 mins until the beans are channeling hot.

STEP 3

Heat the barbecue to tall and toast the bread cuts for 3-5 mins. Beat with the beans and grated cheese, and pop beneath the barbecue until the cheese is liquefied and bubbling. Sprinkle with a small paprika and serve quickly.

Fixings

2 tbsp vegetable oil or other oil

1 expansive onion, finely chopped

4 garlic cloves, finely chopped

1 tsp smoked paprika, additionally additional for sprinkling

1 tsp ground cumin

chipotle chilli paste, to taste, or utilize chilli flakes (discretionary)

200g can chopped tomatoes or passata

2 x 400g cans beans of your choice (kidney and cannellini work well), depleted and flushed

4-8 cuts dried up bread

150g grated cheddar

Simple crêpes

Strategy

STEP 1

Weigh the flour in an expansive container or bowl. Break within the eggs, include half the drain and a squeeze of salt. Whisk to a smooth, thick hitter. Include the remaining milk and whisk once more. Set aside for at slightest 30 mins.

STEP 2

Warm an expansive non-stick crêpe container or singing container. Include a sprinkle of oil, then wipe out the abundance with kitchen paper. When the dish is hot, add sufficient hitter to fair cover the surface, whirling it and pouring any abundance back into the bowl. The flapjack ought to be as lean as conceivable. When the edges are peeling absent from the sides of the skillet, shake it to see in the event that the hotcake effortlessly discharges and is browning on the underside. In case not, cook a small longer. Flip and cook the other side for a miniature or two. Serve, or keep warm in a moo stove.

Fixings

175g plain flour

3 expansive eggs

450ml drain

sunflower oil, for searing

How to poach an egg

Method

STEP 1

Fill a huge pan with water and include the vinegar. As soon as the water begins to bubble, turn the heat down to a stew.

STEP 2

Split the egg into a small bowl. For a culminate egg with no wispy white bits, break into a fine strainer and permit the runnier egg white to deplete off.

STEP 3

Mix the water to make a delicate whirlpool which will offer assistance the egg white wrap around the yolk. At that point carefully slide the egg into the water making beyond any doubt the warm is moo sufficient not to throw the egg around - there ought to as it were being little bubbles rising.

STEP 4

Cook for 3-4 mins, until the white is cooked through.

STEP 5

Evacuate tenderly utilizing an opened spoon and smudge any water from the base on a tea towel or kitchen paper. You can include more than one egg to the dish but make beyond any doubt each one has sufficient room.

Fixings

1 tbsp white wine vinegar

eggs, as many as you need to poach

Our Most Well known Elective

Poached eggs with crushed avocado & tomatoes

**Chocolate-orange French toast
Method**

STEP 1

Warm the stove to 140C/120C fan/gas 1. Cut a take into the side of each thick cut of bread using a little, sharp cut, at that point spoon in a quarter of the marmalade and jab a quarter of the chocolate into each stash.

STEP 2

Whisk the eggs, milk, vanilla, orange pizzazz and cinnamon together in a shallow dish. Dip each cut of bread into the egg blend, making beyond any doubt both sides are completely coated.

STEP 3

Soften ½ tbsp of the butter in a huge broiling dish over a medium warm. Lay a drenched bread cut within the dish and cook until brilliant brown and fresh, almost 2-3 mins per side. Rehash with the remaining cuts. Keep the toasted cuts warm in a low stove whereas cooking the following, including more butter as required.

STEP 4

Put the orange cuts in a skillet with the maple syrup and warm through over a low-medium heat until a few of their juices are discharged. Tidy the French toast with icing sugar and top with the yogurt, orange cuts and warm maple-orange syrup.

Fixings

4 thick cuts of brioche, challah or panettone

2 tbsp jelly

40g dim chocolate, broken into pieces

3 eggs

300ml entirety drain

1 tsp vanilla extract

1 orange, zested, at that point peeled and cut

¼ tsp ground cinnamon

2 tbsp unsalted butter

2 tbsp maple syrup

icing sugar, for cleaning

yogurt or crème fraîche, to serve

Hotcake breakfast tacos

Strategy

STEP 1

Heat the stove to 200C/180C fan/gas 6 and organize the bacon in a single layer on a preparing plate. Heat for 12-14 mins until fresh. In the interim, combine the flour, preparing powder and sugar in a bowl. Whisk the butter, vanilla, drain and egg together in a container. Make a well in the middle of the dry fixings and pour within the damp mixture, whisking to combine. Watch out not to over-whisk – it's fine if there are protuberances.

STEP 2

In a nonstick container, heat a small amount of the oil to a medium temperature. Spoon in 2 tbsp hitter and spread out into a 12cm circle. Cook for 2-3 mins until the edge is set and brilliant. Flip and cook for 1-2 mins more until set. Rehash to create four flapjacks, keeping wrapped up hotcakes warm in a moo stove while you cook the following.

STEP 3

In the interim, for the maple butter, beat the fixings together until smooth. For the mixed eggs, whisk the eggs with a squeeze of salt. Melt the butter in a singing container over a medium warm. Once foaming, pour inside the beaten egg, cook, undisturbed, for 20 seconds, then blend and cook for 1-2 mins more until set, light and delicate. Do not blend as well regularly – you do not need to break up the eggs as well much.

STEP 4

Spread the maple butter over the flapjacks, at that point beat with the eggs, bacon, chives and cheese.

Fixings

100g streaky bacon

125g self-rising flour

1 tsp preparing powder

10g brilliant caster sugar

15g butter, liquefied

1 tsp vanilla extricate

125ml milk

3 egg

½ tbsp neutral-tasting oil

2g chives, finely chopped

30g develop cheddar, grated

For the maple butter

60g butter, mollified

1 tbsp maple syrup

squeeze of ground cinnamon

For the scrambled eggs

2 eggs

1 tbsp butter

Fricasseed bread

Strategy

STEP 1

Warm half the oil or fat in a broiling skillet over a medium-high heat. Once hot, broil the bread for 1 min 30 seconds until brilliant, at that point include the remaining oil or lard, turn the bread over and cook for another 1 min 30 seconds, until golden on both sides.

Fixings

2 tbsp neutral-tasting oil (grapeseed or sunflower work well), or 40g fat

2 cuts thick white bread

Our Most Well known Elective

Pumpkin bread

www.ingramcontent.com/pod-product-compliance
Lightning Source LLC
Chambersburg PA
CBHW062100220526
45471CB00010B/3554